Chair Yoga

by Larry Payne, PhD, and Don Henry

FOREWORD BY Loren Fishman, MD

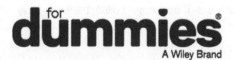

Chair Yoga For Dummies®

Published by: **John Wiley & Sons, Inc.**, 111 River Street, Hoboken, NJ 07030-5774, www.wiley.com

Copyright © 2022 by John Wiley & Sons, Inc., Hoboken, New Jersey

Published simultaneously in Canada

For general information on our other products and services, please contact our Customer Care Department within the U.S. at 877-762-2974, outside the U.S. at 317-572-3993, or fax 317-572-4002. For technical support, please visit https://hub.wiley.com/community/support/dummies.

Wiley publishes in a variety of print and electronic formats and by print-on-demand. Some material included with standard print versions of this book may not be included in e-books or in print-on-demand. If this book refers to media such as a CD or DVD that is not included in the version you purchased, you may download this material at http://booksupport.wiley.com. For more information about Wiley products, visit www.wiley.com.

Library of Congress Control Number: 2022941595

ISBN 978-1-119-88953-3 (pbk); ISBN 978-1-119-88955-7 (ebk); ISBN 978-1-119-88954-0 (ebk)

SKY10073083_041624

Contents at a Glance

Table of Contents

Foreword

Just like Larry Payne — a master Yoga teacher himself — and his co-author, Don Henry, this book about Chair Yoga is smart, easy to understand, and empathetic. Whether you're new to this type of Yoga or not, you will find this book methodically explains what to do and how to do it. It pays attention to your mind first, explaining and giving you the foundation you need not only for Chair Yoga but also for your general health. The meditation it teaches is crucial for Yoga and, in my opinion, for life itself.

Then comes healing stretching for the whole body from the neck down. Every part of the practitioner is subject to meticulous attention. And after that, there is creative thought about actually making Yoga part of a daily routine. The beauty of this is that what is asked of the practitioner is reasonable: first a short 15 minutes, and then more. Without being bound by traditional rules, there is a chapter on how to use weights while doing Chair Yoga. The Yoga itself helps with strength. Add weights, and the benefit is doubled.

Know that you are in excellent hands while reading this book; doing what it recommends undoubtedly adds to health and well-being.

—Dr. Loren Fishman

Introduction

You can find a wide array of Yoga "flavors" in books and even your neighborhood studios. Chair Yoga is just another type, but it's not some trend created for modern audiences. Its roots actually reach into Yoga tradition. Chairs have historically been used as props in Yoga classes, often to

>> Help practitioners get more deeply into a pose

>> Provide a degree of safety by helping with balance or stability or by simply bringing the floor up closer

The great Yoga master, B.K.S. Iyengar, enthusiastically promoted using a chair in order to help his students experience more challenging postures with more security or support. Back in the 1980s, **Lakshmi Voelker** brought the idea of using a chair to America, making Yoga more accessible and even more therapeutic. And co-author Larry Payne dedicated a section of the first edition of *Yoga For Dummies* (Wiley) to Chair Yoga back in 1999.

Make no mistake about it: Chair Yoga is an effective way for you to experience the benefits of practicing Yoga in a way that may make it more accessible to you. Whether it's because of injury or age, your travel schedule, or your work routine, sometimes being able to do Yoga from a chair just makes more sense. And for some people, that accessibility makes all the difference in the world — the difference between actually practicing Yoga or abandoning it altogether.

About This Book

As *Chair Yoga For Dummies* demonstrates, you can readily adopt Yoga as part of your self-care routine, right from your chair.

In this book, we try to offer you a digestible series of poses or movements, not an encyclopedia of all possible postures. The fact is that you can adapt almost any Yoga pose done on a mat to a chair.

Here, we present some of the best and most popular Chair Yoga poses and movements (with about 200 photos) and also incorporate those movements into some sample routines you can do anywhere you find yourself sitting. *Chair Yoga For Dummies* is a great place to try out Yoga or to allow your existing Yoga practice to evolve right along with your body.

In addition to focusing on your muscles and bones, Chair Yoga also gives you an opportunity to nurture your mind. While there may be no one perfect approach to meditation, some form may be just what you need to help reduce stress. (And we all have too much stress, right?) This book dedicates a whole chapter to some of the most straightforward ways to meditate — an activity that's easily performed and easily integrated into Chair Yoga.

Finally, while the book focuses on both the physical and mental benefits of Chair Yoga, it also highlights some vital breath work that can actually benefit both. Like meditation, breathing exercises are an essential part of a Yoga practice, and a chair may be the best place to perform those exercises.

Foolish Assumptions

As we were writing this book, we made a few assumptions about you, dear reader First, we're guessing that you have very good reasons for not pursuing a regular Yoga routine. In reality, however, those reasons are far from being very good— and this book will hopefully prove just that. Maybe you think you're too old or too inflexible. Perhaps you think you're too overweight or too injured. And secondly, if you're still looking for an excuse, there's always that onerous lack of free time or appropriate space. Our guess — our assumption — is you might be clinging to one or more of these "very good reasons."

Of course, if you happen to be a super-flexible former gymnast (or maybe just an average 16-year-old), you may need to find the full, traditional expression of a particular Yoga pose simply to feel a stretch. If, however, your flexibility is more limited than that, you don't have to go as deeply into a pose in order to feel the exact same degree of stretch or strengthening. Your so-called limitation may indeed be due to injury, inexperience, age, weight, or even workload. Or maybe you just (gasp!) have an average range of motion. The goal of a Yoga practice should be improved physical and mental health, so put less focus on what it looks like and more on what it's doing for your body and mind. And Chair Yoga can do a lot.

Icons Used in This Book

We use several icons throughout this book to help you better navigate the text and find the most important and helpful bits:

TIP

This icon identifies special suggestions that you may want to keep in mind as you practice a Chair Yoga routine or try a pose.

REMEMBER

Some things are worth keeping in mind, particularly when attempting a new posture or trying a new routine.

WARNING

Even Chair Yoga, as accommodating as it attempts to be, can lead to injury if you're not mindful. These paragraphs may help you to pay attention to certain obstacles, but they in no way substitute for the good advice of your doctor or other health care practitioner.

TECHNICAL STUFF

Text marked with a Technical Stuff icon is interesting (we like to think), but ultimately it isn't essential for getting a handle on Chair Yoga. If you want to get in and get out, you can skip these bits without compromising your understanding of the topic.

Beyond the Book

An effective way to focus on some of the key concepts of this book is to check out the online Cheat Sheet that summarizes many of the important takeaways relating to a Chair Yoga practice. Go online to dummies.com and search for **Chair Yoga For Dummies Cheat Sheet.**

Where to Go from Here

If you want a complete picture of Chair Yoga, you can definitely read this book straight through. But you don't have to go cover to cover to meet your needs.

Want to target a specific part or parts of your body? Try the chapters in Part 2. Need a premade Chair Yoga routine for your busy schedule? Chapters 16 and 17 can help. Just looking for some tips on mindful breathing? Exhale and flip to Chapter 3. However you read this book, remember that Yoga — including Chair Yoga — needs to serve you, not the other way around.

1

Yoga for Life

IN THIS PART . . .

Uncover the health benefits of simple movements.

Consider what kind of teaching you want and how to prepare your Chair Yoga practice area.

Discover the power of your breath.

Review how meditation can have a profound impact on your mental fitness.

Chapter **1**

Checking Out Chair Yoga

Getting up and down off the floor or a Yoga mat can be a challenge for some people. But no one should be left off the Yoga bandwagon.

REMEMBER

For any number of reasons, you may choose to practice Yoga while sitting in a chair. Chair Yoga doesn't require that up-and-down flow you may find in other Yoga classes. You can remain in a seated position where you feel more stable — even safer — while still reaping some of Yoga's most significant benefits:

>> More flexibility

>> Increased strength

>> Better balance

>> Improved circulation

>> Decreased anxiety and stress

>> Reduced pain

>> Better sleep

>> Greater willpower

These benefits have been acknowledged over the years by not only Yoga teachers and students but also Western medicine itself.

Chair Yoga is just one approach or technique, but it may in fact be the smartest one. The key to making your movements truly Yogic is to synchronize them with your breath. That coordination keeps you relaxed and allows your body to benefit from the power of simple movements.

Harnessing the Power of Simple Movements

Sitting in front of a screen or in a line of slow-moving commuter traffic can render you relatively motionless for hours at a time. In fact, health practioners often warn about how being sedentary, especially sitting too much, is actually almost the same threat to good health as smoking is.

Yoga teachers and Yoga therapists alike talk about how much you can gain from the simplest of movements.Simple and safe movements can

>> Build muscle strength

>> Increase flexibility

>> Increase bone density (in some practitioners)

>> Lubricate your joints

>> Improve your will power

>> Decrease anxiety and stress

>> Exercise your heart and lungs

You can read more about some of these benefits in the following section.

The ultimate objective is to avoid inactivity but, at the same time, proceed both slowly and thoughtfully. That's where Chair Yoga comes in. Although you can move in many ways, Chair Yoga may be both the perfect and the safest activity. It's also a great way to supplement other aerobic and strength training exercises.

If you want to hang on to a Yoga practice but find your body is making new demands, consider Chair Yoga. If you're new to Yoga and maybe feel too old or too inflexible, this approach may be an ideal entry point.

At the end of the day, Yoga — even Chair Yoga — needs to make you feel better. Listen to your body, don't allow yourself to endure pain, and most of all, have fun!

When a Yoga Mat Just Doesn't Work

The chair has a long history in Yoga. It's a traditional prop, often used for safety and support in the pursuit of the classic form of a pose. Great Yoga masters like B.K.S. Iyengar employed the chair by using innovative methods to help students move into otherwise difficult postures.

But Chair Yoga is something different. Popularized in the USA by Lakshmi Voelker back in the 1980s, it's more about making Yoga accessible to everyone. It's about finding ways for Yoga to accommodate the particular needs of the practitioner rather than finding ways for the practitioner to adapt to a pose. Chair Yoga is about practicing in a way that serves your fitness goals and makes you want to come back again and again.

Seniors need Yoga, too

Without a doubt, many senior centers have mat Yoga classes that are well attended by people in their '60s, '70s, and even '80s. These people use their mats in the traditional way, which means they get up and down off the floor at various points throughout the class. Some seniors, however, just can't do that. Chair Yoga provides an alternative for almost anyone.

REMEMBER

Your body changes as you get older, and you may lose certain capabilities. Even in an average Yoga class, practitioners can't do the things they did when they were younger — at least not without the risk of getting injured.

Deskbound employees

Whether they're self-imposed or handed down by an employer, productivity demands can keep you at a desk for too many hours at a time. (Of course, many people willingly sit in front of their computers for extended periods of time, oblivious to the clock and the rest of the world around them.)

Chair Yoga provides a way to counteract all the negative aspects of sitting at a desk for long periods of time and receive the benefits of thoughtful movements without leaving the desk chair.

Leaving on a jet plane

If you find yourself sitting for long periods of time on an airplane, watching an in-flight movie or even splurging on a cocktail often just isn't enough to help you relax or bring the circulation back into your limbs. And space is always an issue on a plane.

These are some of the challenges faced by the frequent traveler. Chair Yoga can certainly offer relief to the tight and tense traveler

Yoga for expecting moms

WARNING

All expecting mothers need to talk with their obstetricians about doing exercise. Knowing the things you should look out for or avoid entirely is critical.

This book doesn't deal specifically with prenatal Yoga. Chair Yoga, however, does offer the expecting mother some distinct advantages. Specifically, using the chair as a prop can help support body weight as well as bring the stability of the floor up higher.

The goal, of course, is to avoid any kind of pressure on the abdomen (including certain kinds of twisting), so listen to your body and your doctor when it comes to doing any physical activity — even Chair Yoga. Then, select the poses and movements you think would be beneficial.

The good news is that expecting mothers can certainly practice both breathwork and meditation from the comfort of their chairs. Both can reduce or eliminate stress and pain in your mind and your body.

Practicing yoga when you have limited mobility

Even people who have athletic Yoga practices find their abilities are constrained or deactivated from time to time. This typically occurs as the result of injury or illness. Chair Yoga is often a way for these people to keep practicing even though their range of motion is temporarily limited.

If this is you, be mindful of any warnings that may come from your doctor. But also remember that Chair Yoga is almost always a better alternative to complete immobility. A thoughtful practitioner can keep some parts of their body limber while allowing other parts to heal.

Enjoying the Benefits of Yoga

If you look at Yoga as more of a healing activity rather than simply a process of bringing your body into super-flexible poses, then the mental and physical benefits derived from a Yoga practice are definitely more important than how it may "look."

As we note earlier in the chapter, even Western medicine recognizes the power of Yoga, and Chair Yoga offers most of the same benefits.

Moving feels good

"Sitting is the new smoking" has almost reached the status of being a cliché, but it still resonates loudly. The impact of too much sitting — of too much inactivity — takes a toll on both your body and your spirit. Clearly, moving makes you feel better.

The implication here is pretty straightforward. If you're currently not moving around enough, adding Chair Yoga as a regular routine will yield returns. You may not readily see them initially, but they'll ultimately become wonderfully apparent.

Working the joints

Just by doing some of the most basic movements in Chair Yoga, you keep your joints mobile and well lubricated. The key is to not overdo it, so always listen to what your body's saying and stop moving when it's time.

Anyone can benefit from good joint health, but if you happen to have arthritis, you may discover some particular relief associated with certain movements. Some arthritic pain, for example, comes from joint stiffness, so movements that reinforce mobility and range-of-motion can help. Check out Part 2 for Chair Yoga movements that target the joints.

Stretching and strengthening the muscles

In general, Yoga contributes to muscle health in many ways. By adding Chair Yoga to your routine (or using Chair Yoga to continue your already established Yoga practice) you may be building muscle, maintaining and expanding your flexibility, and even improving your balance as you strengthen the muscles responsible for it.

Although not every Yoga movement is intended to build muscle, some movements and poses do achieve that. Perhaps you hold a pose to build strength or perform several repetitions (it's amazing how even the simplest movement can be challenging after a few reps).

Building some bone

Research tends to suggest that Yoga can increase bone density. This not only is important for anyone wanting healthy bones but also has compelling implications for those with osteoporosis-related diseases or those trying to prevent those types of conditions. (Loren Fishman, MD, who wrote the Foreword to this book, has done some extensive work on this subject.)

REMEMBER

Researchers don't know yet whether Chair Yoga automatically increases bone density; however, movements that involve using body weight to build muscle, improve circulation, or even create a better attitude may ultimately help build healthier bones.

Relieving stress and anxiety

Stress just seems to be a given. Whether it's from work, a family situation, or something else, you can probably point to any number of things that bring stress or anxiety into your life. As of this writing, the ongoing COVID-19 pandemic certainly has brought a degree of anxiety into everyone's life.

Chair Yoga offers enough gentle movement that it actually counteracts the impacts of stress. Even if you practice for only for 15 minutes, if you're focusing your attention on some movement or pose, your mind forgets (for a while, anyway) anything that's causing you stress or worry.

TIP

In addition to helping you stay stretched out and mobile, Chair Yoga can also reduce tension through breathing exercises and meditation — two extremely beneficial activities you can do in your chair just about anywhere.

Giving Chair Yoga a Try

Try the following movements while using any chair — though chosing a chair without wheels or a swivel function is highly recommended in order to prevent the chair from unwanted movement. The purpose of introducing a couple of routines in Chapter 1 is to show you just how easily you can do Chair Yoga almost anywhere and how it often uses simple movements that ultimately give you a lot of bang for your buck.

Cross/crawl patterning

The cross/crawl patterning routine may seem on the surface to be a very simple movement — and it probably is. Yet applying this concept to fitness training is a very old approach. It begins to stretch out some of the muscles in your shoulders and hips and also moves and lubricates some of the joints.

In addition, cross/crawl patterning not only requires that opposite sides of your body work in coordination but also makes similar demands on your mind. The right and left hemispheres of the brain have to effectively communicate with one another.

In the following routine, we've adapted the classic cross/crawl patterning to the chair:

1. **Find a chair and have a seat.**

   This chair may be one you use on an ongoing basis, so selecting something without arms will give you more room.

2. **Sit upright, being mindful of your posture; your arms can hang straight at your side (see Figure 1-1).**

   Even in the chair, you can focus on maintaining good posture. Doing so positions your lungs and diaphragm to function more freely. Think about lining up your ears right above your shoulders and keeping your shoulders directly above your hips. Your feet should be flat on the ground.

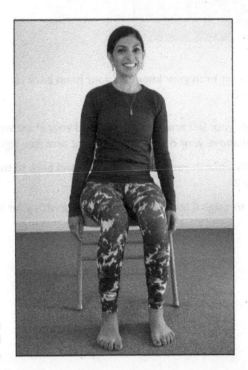

FIGURE 1-1:
Sitting with good posture.

3. On an inhale, lift your right knee upward toward your chest while raising your left hand above your head with a straight arm (see Figure 1-2).

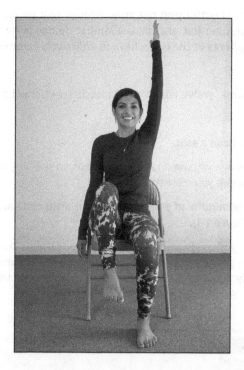

FIGURE 1-2:
Lifting your arm
and leg.

4. Exhale as you lower both your knee and your hand back to the starting position in Step 2.

5. On an inhale, lift your left knee upward toward your chest while raising your right hand above your head with a straight arm (see Figure 1-3).

6. Exhale as you lower both your knee and your hand back to the starting position in Step 2.

7. Repeat Steps 2 through 6 five more times, moving with your breath.

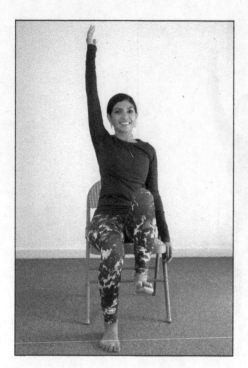

FIGURE 1-3:
Doing the
other side.

Seated rejuvenation sequence

This flowing sequence is a variation of the Rejuvenation Sequence created by coauthor Larry Payne for Prime of Life Yoga. It's essentially a type of *sun salutation*, a moving sequence traditionally done in the morning, perhaps as part of a morning ritual. From a more modern perspective, this routine is a great way to warm up your entire body before continuing on with your practice.

1. Sit upright in your chair and open your legs to about hip width.

2. Let your arms hang straight down at your sides.

3. As you inhale, sweep your straight arms out to the side and bring them over your head with your palms facing (see Figure 1-4).

4. As you exhale, bring your straight arms down on the outside of your legs and fold over, allowing your head to drop between your legs (see Figure 1-5).

If you have any issues that dropping your head may exacerbate, only bend down halfway, keeping your hands on your thighs.

TIP

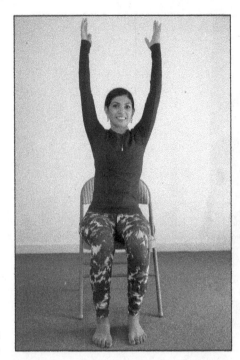

FIGURE 1-4:
Reaching up.

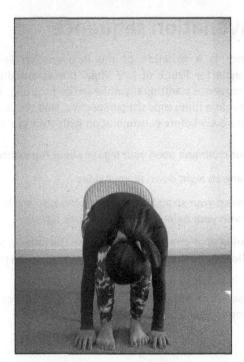

FIGURE 1-5:
Folding forward.

5. As you inhale, raise your torso halfway up so your back is flat and parallel to the ground and spread your arms straight out to the sides (see Figure 1-6).

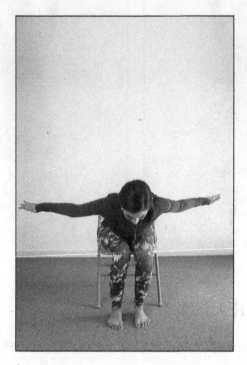

FIGURE 1-6: Halfway up.

6. On an exhale, drop your head and arms back to the forward fold as in Step 4.

7. On an inhale, reach up as you come into a squat just off of your chair (see Figure 1-7b).

   Alternatively, you can stay seated as you reach up, pressing your feet into the ground as shown in Figure 1-7a.

8. On an exhale, come back to the starting position from Step 2, sitting tall in your seat with your arms dropped to the side.

9. Repeat Steps 1 through 8 four to six times.

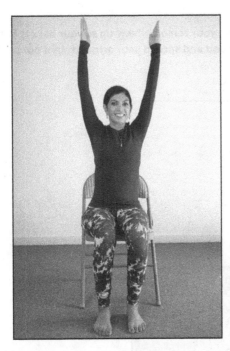 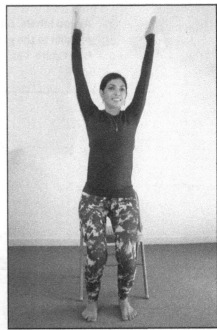

FIGURE 1-7:
Seated or in a
squat.

CHERISH THE CHAIR

The great Yoga master, B.K.S. Iyengar, is famous for using props when teaching Yoga — and Iyengar Yoga uses chairs in very creative ways. Chairs often provide support to practitioners who need help getting into more demanding postures.

Co-author Larry Payne is intimately aware of this style of Yoga because he studied with Iyengar while in India. He recalls that, much to the chagrin of many local students, Iyengar was sometimes referred to as "the furniture Yogi" because of his use of so many different props.

But don't think Iyengar was offering some watered-down version of Yoga — even if he did allow his students to use props. Iyengar Yoga is, in fact, extremely demanding, usually striving toward the classic pose but sometimes using a chair to not only get there but also stay there longer.

Of course, the Chair Yoga described in this book is much more accessible. You should be able to perform some version of these postures and movements regardless of your physical challenges, age, flexibility, or experience. Still, it's worth noting that long before a chair was used to make Yoga more accessible to anyone, it was no stranger to a Yoga studio — and any Yoga student should welcome the sight of a chair.

Chapter **2**

Getting Ready for Chair Yoga

I f you're considering Chair Yoga as a way to cultivate better physical and mental fitness, you don't really have to do a lot to prepare to jump right in. You don't need to buy expensive equipment, you don't need a uniform or flashy outfit, and you don't even need a team or partner. Just a comfy chair and a good attitude will set you on the pathway to success.

However, you still have to make a few decisions along the way, and this chapter helps address those choices. Just know that whatever you decide, you can still access — and even enhance — Yoga's benefits by adding a chair to the equation.

Deciding on the Guidance That Works for You

Picking the source or sources you want to use to continue your Chair Yoga education is certainly an important choice. The following sections explore some of the options available to you.

Attending real-time classes

One of the most obvious advantages of in-person Chair Yoga is that you're part of a community. You're learning and practicing with people who share your desire to do Yoga in a chair. The social component involved in going to a studio, sitting in your chair next to other people in chairs, and getting their support and encouragement adds additional health benefits.

What's probably more important, however, is the fact that your teacher is right there keeping you as safe as possible. Because the teacher's eyes are on you, they can learn about your practice and your body and perhaps suggest particular poses or modifications that serve your specific needs. A real-time chair class not only keeps you safer but probably also allows you to progress more quickly.

The downside is that you have to leave the comfort of your home and travel to a studio — one that offers Chair Yoga classes at a convenient time.

REMEMBER

These days, you undoubtedly have the option of attending a virtual class on a platform like Zoom or Microsoft Teams. These types of classes are still real-time classes. You're still practicing with other students, and the teacher can keep an eye on you, albiet over video. (Of course, in the virtual world, you have control over how much anybody sees.)

Following videos on your own time

A video can be a great way to learn something, particularly because you can hear a lecture and see a demonstration at the same time. After all, video is a visual medium.

If you have access to a site like YouTube, you can probably find hundreds of Chair Yoga videos available to you at no cost. But that bargain can be both a blessing and a curse. The sheer quantity of videos available to you means you have to sort through all of the options and try to discern what video and what teacher will serve your particular needs.

WARNING

Unfortunately, not all teachers are good, and not all videos will protect you from injury. So be thoughful in your selection — and be prepared to put up with some commercials.

Pursuing a practice with books

Because you're already reading this work, you've most likely decided that books are one way you plan on finding more information about Chair Yoga. Chances are you'll rely on more than one. That's why they make bookshelves, right?

Books allow you to take in information at your own speed and can also provide a visual component with illustrations and photographs. A detailed, well-illustrated Chair Yoga book (like this one, for example) is a great way to discover more about the practice.

REMEMBER

Literally anyone can upload a video to the Internet (see the preceding section), but having a book come from a legitimate publisher is a much more vetted process. If your starting point is a well-known publisher or author, you're certainly ahead of the game.

Making Preparations

Chair Yoga is something you can do anywhere at any time, but establishing a regular routine may be easier if you do a little bit of preparing first. Even the smallest efforts upfront pay off big-time down the road.

The secret to success is to do Chair Yoga with consistency. That's why doing some planning ahead is worthwhile.

Talking to your health care provider

REMEMBER

Whether you're dealing with an illness, recovering from an injury, or even feeling just fine, you should always talk to your doctor before beginning any exercise program, including Chair Yoga. This book helps prepare you to have a conversation about what Chair Yoga entails, and your doctor or other health care provider can tell you whether you should avoid any certain postures or movements.

If nothing else, getting a thumbs-up to proceed with your practice should give you a sense of security that may make your Chair Yoga experience that much more enjoyable.

Scoping out your space

If you're going to reap the benefits of practicing Yoga, you need to do it on a regular basis and not just sporadically. With that in mind, identify a place — perhaps somewhere right in your home — that you can go to every day to do your Chair Yoga. Make it a routine, like brushing your teeth.

One of the advantages of this type of Yoga is that you don't need a lot of space. But you do want to select a location that allows you to reach your arms up and out. Even if you're in a studio class, make sure the people around you aren't so close that they restrict your movement in any way. As you pick up the chair versions of various poses, you can chose what suits both your body and your space.

Knowing what to wear

In general, Yoga shouldn't be about the clothes. You don't need to go to a high-end Yoga store to find the latest in studio fashion. Yet you do want to consider some practicalities:

>> **Freedom of movement:** Wear clothing that lets you bend, stretch, and reach for the sky. If you're wearing something that makes any of these movements more difficult, it's probably not the best Chair Yoga ensemble.

>> **Your modesty needs:** Many of the movements and postures in Chair Yoga are a bit exaggerated — definitely not what most people typically do in everyday life. If you find that your shirt rides up or your waistband tends to inch down, you may want to choose something else to wear.

You definitely don't want to feel restricted or self-conscious, nor do you want to instill those feelings in others if you're in a group class.

Finding a Chair for Your Derriere

You don't have to go out and buy a special chair in order to do Chair Yoga. That extra chair sitting in your guest room may be just perfect. The important thing is to be comfortable. Perhaps the biggest thing to consider is finding a chair without arms, only because arms can sometimes get in the way of your movements.

Think of your chair as your partner — or maybe as your Yoga mat. You'll work together to find the most beneficial expressions of poses and movements. Be sure you select a chair in which you enjoy sitting.

Note: Since you're looking for a chair that will give you a sense of stability, avoid chairs on wheels or that swivel. You should be the only one moving in these routines, not your chair.

Snagging a sturdy seat

You definitely won't find comfort in a chair that feels wobbly, so take the time to select a chair that's both comfortable and safe. That way, you can move in and out of poses more confidently and may even feel comfortable closing your eyes, something that can be useful in simply relaxing.

For extra support, you can place the chair with its back legs up against a wall as shown in Figure 2-1. This setup can be particularly useful for expecting mothers, seniors, or anyone concerned about the chair sliding or even tipping backward.

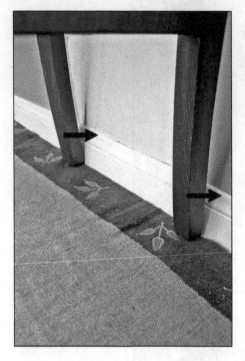

Your chair is going to be your only partner and your best source of support, so chose it carefully. Of course, you can always have another chair nearby if you need additional support getting up and down, and older practitioners may want to keep their canes or walkers within arm's reach.

Preventing your feet from dangling

Not all chairs are created equal. For example, they can vary in height, which may be problematic. Often, especially if you're under five feet, five inches tall, your feet can actually dangle toward the ground as Figure 2-2 illustrates. That's simply not good for your back.

If you can't find a chair that is just the right height, put something underneath your feet to level them off like in Figure 2-3. A Yoga block or even a folded blanket may be what you need. Whatever you use, your back will thank you for it.

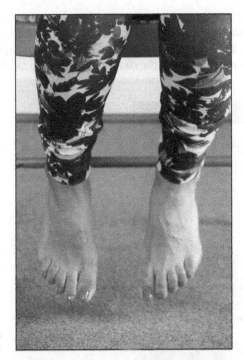

FIGURE 2-2:
Dangling feet.

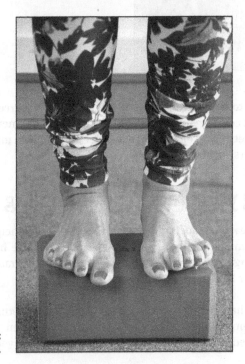

FIGURE 2-3:
Feet on a block.

Setting Aside Time to Sit and Get Fit

Sometimes a busy schedule can overshadow even the most enjoyable activities in life. That's why setting aside a specific time in your daily or weekly routine to dedicate to Chair Yoga is important. If you don't make it part of your life, it'll remain on the periphery, along with all the related fitness and stress reduction benefits.

TIP

If a daily practice seems too much for now, start with a weekly routine. After your body and mind experience the nurturing Chair Yoga can offer, you can always increase the frequency of your routines. Whether you're working from your home or attending class nearby, setting aside a specific time in your schedule will lead to better and faster results.

You can start with the routines at the end of this book. We offer 15-minute and 30-minute routines for both beginners and more advanced Yogis. Both of these durations work well at home. If you decide to attend a group class, plan on spending about one hour.

Don't overestimate the amount of time you can dedicate to Chair Yoga. Life always has a way of interfering with noblest of intentions. The good news is you can accomplish a lot — even if you only have 15 minutes.

Taking a Test Run in Your Chair

Before you begin your exploration of Chair Yoga, you need to check a couple of things:

>> The difference between a comfortable seated position and a strong-posture position, which better facilitates your breathing

>> The height of your chair (and dealing with any dangling)

The following simple routine should adequately check out both these things.

1. **Sit in your chair and choose any position that's comfortable.**

   When you start practicing, you won't be in this casual pose, but for now feel free to sit back against the chair and even cross your legs.

2. **Move into a more upright position by sliding forward, leaving some space behind you and making sure your feet are on the floor; sit tall with your ears over your shoulders and your shoulders over your hips (see Figure 2-4).**

   Note your upright posture and how this position may differ from the more casual position you had in Step 1.

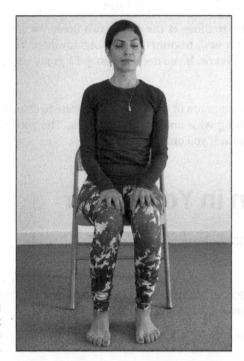

FIGURE 2-4:
An upright posture in the chair.

TIP

If your feet don't touch the ground even after you slide forward, your chair is probably too tall. You can try another chair or use props to bring the floor up to you, as we describe in the earlier section "Preventing your feet from dangling."

AN EYE ON COMPLIANCE

Talk to any health or wellness professional and one of the biggest challenges they face is "patient compliance." Even when we know what's good for us, all too often it's just difficult to comply. That goes for taking medicine, making dietary changes, performing rehab exercises — and yes, even doing Chair Yoga.

As you contemplate practicing Yoga from a chair, be realistic about the amount of time you can dedicate to it. For example, pledging to yourself 15 minutes a day and then doing it is infinitely better than promising one hour a day and then not doing it (for whatever reason). While things are always going to come up, you ultimately want to feel like you're truly making an effort.

Of course, there's a long list of reasons why sticking to a regular Chair Yoga program can be challenging. Perhaps you have an erratic work schedule, or your physical condition makes it easy to justify skipping a day. Try to make these types of obstacles more the exception than the rule.

This book already talks about setting aside time for Chair Yoga, but the biggest challenge in Chair Yoga is not the twisting poses or stretching movements. It's consistency — and that is your primary pathway to better health.

Chapter 3

Inhale, Exhale: Controlling Your Breath

The power of your own breath is something you should learn to harness. It may be one of the most useful tools in your personal tool kit; it's that important.

REMEMBER

Some of the benefits associated with controlling your breath include the following:

>> Managing your pain

>> Lessening your stress level

>> Slowing your heart rate

>> Building basic energy

>> Improving your digestive processes

>> Triggering the production of endorphins

>> Encouraging good posture

>> Improving your sleep

We put this breathing chapter right up front because, as critical as your breath may be to your overall health, it is also easily forgotten when you start to focus your attention on the poses and movements. Of course, those poses and movements are only effective when they're thoughtfully coordinated with your breath. Any good Yoga teacher will remind you of that — over and over again. And this chapter explains why breathing is also an essential part of Chair Yoga.

Understanding Why Breathing Is Important in Yoga

Yoga seems to put a great deal of focus on the breath, and Chair Yoga is no different. The goal is to breathe in such a way that the body remains as relaxed as possible even during strenuous movement.

REMEMBER

Most Yogic traditions see the practice of breath work (*pranayama*) as being just as important as the postures themselves (*asana*) are. Some Yogis would even say that it's more important.

Even the most ancient Yogic texts recognize the importance of breathing in the pursuit of physical health and emotional well-being. Indeed, Yoga recognizes a link among body, breath, and mind and works to make you more aware of that link during your practice.

Connecting good breathing and good posture

Breathing and good health are directly correlated, and not just because your breathing brings necessary oxygen into your body. When you breathe — especially when you breathe deeply — you may in fact be improving your overall posture.

>> Your *intercostal muscles* (the muscles between your ribs) and rib cage keep their form and flexibility instead of collapsing.

>> A deep breath elongates your spine and actually maintains the space between your vertabrae while reducing the pressure on the front of them.

>> You may also support the natural curves of your spine, potentially reducing any tension or stress you're carrying in your spine.

Sending a message to relax

Think about it: When you're in trouble, your breathing speeds up, probably short-ens, and becomes shallow. On the other hand, a state of relaxation may very well conincide with easy, deep breathing. By consciously adapting that slow breathing pattern, you send a message to your brain, to your parasympathetic nervous sys-tem, that you can relax.

REMEMBER

The *parasympathetic nervous system* is the part of your autonomic nevous system that regulates your ability to relax. The *sympathetic nevous system* regulates the fight-or-flight response.

Most of the time, the goal is to trigger relaxation — to destress — and you can do that with some slow, deep breathing.

Extending your exhale

Over and over again, traditional Yoga philosophy advocates the idea of extending the exhale. In fact, in Sutra 1.34 of the *Yoga Sutras* (a philisophical composition on which much of Yoga is based), Patanjali says, "The practice of breathing exercises involving extended exhalation might be helpful." (This is from the TKV Desikachar translation.)

SENDING YOU OFF TO DREAMLAND

The potential negative effects of not getting enough sleep are certainly something to consider. They include impaired job productivity, diminished academic performance, and health risks like high blood pressure, heart disease, and even obesity.

Sleep disorders and stress do seem to be directly correlated. Breathing exercises, the kind you can do in Chair Yoga, may actually help. In fact, you can probably make a strong argument that most Yoga practices are a good way to address issues like insomnia.

To that end, Yoga experts who focus on breath work would say that most routines are specifically designed to reduce stress and anxiety. Breathing exercises give the mind something to focus on besides the day-to-day demands of work, parenting, and so on. So although any of that can keep you up at night, breath work may make falling asleep and staying asleep easier.

Extending the exhale simply means to make your exhale longer than your inhale. Singers do it all the time when they want to sing a long note; wind instrumentalists probably do, too. By only letting air out a little at a time, you're sustaining — extending — that exhale.

REMEMBER

Some breathing exercises specifically ask you to extend your exhale. But even without specific instructions, make this extension your goal. Extended exhales help you connect to the parasympathetic nervous system and ultimately to greater relaxation.

Breathing with postures: A moving meditation

Coordinating your breath with movement is an essential part of any type of Yoga. The union of your breath, mind, and body is at the heart of a Yoga practice and is what distinguishes Yoga from other forms of movement and exercise.

Consider these two essential aspects of a moving meditation:

>> Moving with your breath

>> Focusing your thoughts on the movement

Sometimes, all the breath cues in Yoga can be irritating: inhale here, exhale there. Yet some positions are easier to hold when breathing in a certain way. A forward fold, for example, is more accessible on an exhale, when your diaphragm returns to the top of your abdominal cavity, up and out of the way. You can bend more deeply.

In Yoga, the expression of this idea is quite straightforward: When the body opens, you usually inhale. When the bodyfolds, you usually exhale. Allowing your breath to move with your body allows you to focus on the movement, stay in the present, and think about the pose rather than your grocery list. And if you maintain that focus, your body, breath, and mind are all working together in a moving meditation.

Focusing on the Body Parts Used in Breathing

The breath process involves various parts of the body (don't worry; we're not going to give you a full-blown anatomy lesson here):

- » Nose
- » Mouth
- » Throat
- » Larynx
- » Trachea (often called the windpipe)
- » Ribs
- » Bronchial airways
- » Diaphragm
- » Lungs

The job of all these parts, working together, is to take in oxygen (to nourish the rest of the body) and to expel carbon dioxide. Both your ribs and your diaphragm help bring air in and out of your lungs.

REMEMBER

Note the body parts that *aren't* listed here. Your shoulders, for example, should have nothing to do with the relaxed breathing process and shouldn't move a lot with your inhales and exhales. (This may not be true in more rigorous breathing or if you're dealing with respiratory ailments like chronic obstructive pulmonary disease [COPD] or emphysema.)

For the most part, you should be breathing exclusively through your nose. This concept is an important one in Yoga and really makes a lot of sense:

- » Your nasal passages are much smaller than your gaping mouth, which requires your breathing to be slower.
- » The hairs in your nasal passages filter the air you bring into your body.
- » Inhaling through the nose also warms and moistens the air before it reaches your lungs.

In other words, acknowledging the Indian tradition, your nose is for breathing; your mouth is for eating.

REMEMBER

Of course, you always want to minimize stress. If you need to breathe through your mouth (maybe you have a cold, allergies, or a medical condition that prevents easy nose breathing), by all means do.

Dealing with Breathing Problems

The various Chair Yoga poses themselves stretch and strengthen muscles that support the expansion and contraction of the lungs (inhaling and exhaling) and the movement of the diaphragm.

TIP

Having said that, breathing routines typically do the same thing. Taking deep breaths is the key to keeping your lungs healthy. Typical breathing problems that may benefit from regular breath work include these:

>> COPD

>> Asthma

>> Bronchitis

>> Emphysema

Breath work typically accomplishes the following:

>> Expands lung capacity with more air

>> Reduces stress

>> Slows the breath rate

>> Increases circulation

>> Eliminates waste products (on the exhale)

>> Allows your focus to turn inward

Turning to Your Breathing to Manage Stress and Pain

The benefits of breath work are numerous, although how much any of these techniques reduces stress and even chronic pain varies from person to person. Breathing exercises don't come with a money-back guarantee. But the potential for positive results is too important not to pursue. Most Yoga therapists, based on working with patients who deal with stress and chronic pain, see breath work as a powerful place to start.

For people who do suffer with chronic pain often find it involves a stress component. By reducing your stress level, you cause your body to relax, often reducing the degree of pain.

Of course, people in pain also tend to move less, which can lead to stiffness and more pain. Not only does a Chair Yoga practice provide the necessary movement and stretching, but it also offers the opportunity to practice the breath work designed to keep your respiratory system healthy and decrease the tension that often exacerbates pain.

Focus breathing

Too often, you may find that you're taking quick, shallow breaths. Your brain interpets that as a sign that you're in some kind of trouble. To be of help, your bloodstream is flooded with hormones like adrenaline or cortisol (the stress hormone) to help you stay and fight your way out of trouble, or maybe just to run away. That shallow breathing pattern, however, is probably just a bad habit.

The focus breathing exercise described here will have the opposite effect. Not only does it help you to relax, but it may even lower your blood pressure and heart rate.

Of course, breathing is something you've been doing, pretty much without thinking, since the first moment you were born. No matter how you breathe, trying to change it now can be somewhat annoying, even challenging, for some people.

If some of the breathing routines recommended in this book (or perhaps routines that you discover elsewhere) seem too challenging, focus breathing is a great place to start. Even this simple technique can help you relax and distract you from chronic pain.

A renowned respiratory therapist once observed that his patients who had the hardest time changing the way they breathe were Yoga teachers. Perhaps that's exactly right because Yogis spend so much time learning to control their breath that they have a hard time going back. But now it's your turn to change your breathing — to face the challenge but hopefully to also reap the rewards.

To practice focus breathing, following these steps:

1. Sit upright in your chair with your head over your shoulders.

2. Place your left hand on your stomach and your right hand on your chest as shown in Figure 3-1.

3. **Inhale deeply through your nose and notice where you feel like the air is flowing.**

    Is it more into your stomach? Your chest? Both?

4. **Exhale deeply through your nose.**

5. **Repeat Steps 1 through 4 for a total of six breaths.**

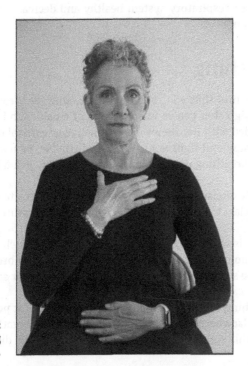

FIGURE 3-1:
Focus breathing
hand positions.

Belly breathing

The *belly breathing* technique asks you to focus on the sensation of your stomach rising and falling as you breathe. This type of breathing is intended to help you relax and maybe even sleep better.

The diaphragm is basically a muscle that helps move air in and out. As you breathe, your diaphragm (that sits underneath your lungs) flattens and moves down toward your abdominal cavity. Your stomach may rise and fall in the breathing process, giving you the sensation that air is actually flowing into your stomach. But we all know that air only flows into the lungs. This technique puts your attention on the movement of your diaphragm. In addition to being good for stress reduction, it may actually provide a sort of massage to parts of the lower back and pelvic floor.

To practice belly breathing, follow these steps:

1. Sit upright in your chair with your head over your shoulders.

2. Place both hands comfortably on your stomach as shown in Figure 3-2.

3. Inhale through your nose, feeling your stomach rise.

4. Exhale through your nose, feeling your stomach deflate.

5. Repeat Steps 1 through 4 for a total of eight breaths.

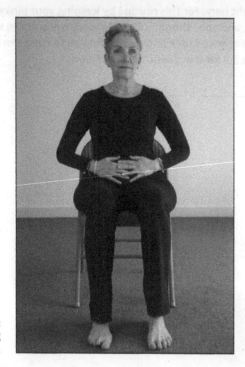

FIGURE 3-2:
Belly breathing
hand positions.

TIP

As you perform this routine, try to keep your chest out of the process. You may even want to put one of your hands on your chest just to be sure it's remaining as still as possible.

Alternate nostril breathing

The goal of *alternate nostril breathing* is to give you yet another way to link your mind with your breath. In this exercise, you inhale and exhale through one nostril at a time rather than two. It requires some concentration to do it, but the benefits include

>> Slower breath rate

>> Better mental focus

>> Reduction of stress

To practice altnerate nostril breathing, follow these steps:

1. **Sit comfortably in your chair with your back straight, your left hand can rest on your left thigh.**

2. **Prepare your right hand for this routine by keeping your pinky finger, your ring finger, and your thumb fully extended, while at the same time bringing the tips of your index and middle fingers to the palm of your hand (see Figure 3-3 for the classic hand position).**

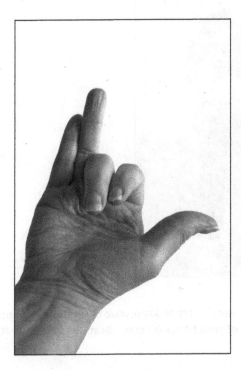

FIGURE 3-3:
Hand position.

3. **Place your right hand so that your thumb is resting lightly on your right nostril, and your little and ring fingers are near your left nostril. Your index and middle fingers are tucked lightly into your hand (near the ball of your thumb).**

4. **Close your right nostril and inhale gently but fully through your left nostril (see Figure 3-4).**

Don't strain.

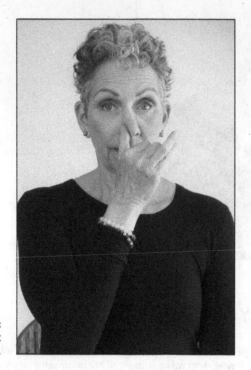

FIGURE 3-4:
Closing your right nostril.

5. **Open your right nostril, close your left nostril with your ring and pinky fingers, and exhale through the open right nostril (see Figure 3-5).**

6. **Inhale through your right nostril and then block it and exhale through your left.**

7. **Repeat Steps 3 through 5 10 to 15 times.**

With practice, you can gradually increase the number of repetitions.

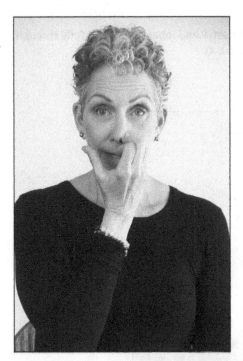

FIGURE 3-5:
Closing your
left nostril.

BE STILL MY HEART

Many people and scholars refer to Tirumalai Krishnamacharya as the "Father of Modern Yoga." Co-author Larry Payne, who was a student of Krishnamacharya's son, met the man while visiting his home in India. Larry can attest, firsthand, to the Yoga Master's formidable presence whenever he entered a room. Krishnamacharya was not only a Yoga teacher with many famous students, he was an ayurvedic specialist with great healing ability and also a true scholar in his own right. He also famously claimed to use breathing and meditation techniques to stop his own heart.

Of course, he wasn't the only Yoga Master to make that assertion, but whether any Yogi can actually stop their heart is one of those East versus West conundrums that's still debated today. And please don't try this at home.

There may be a blend of both science and legend in these stories, but contemporary medicine does indeed acknowledge the relationship between breath and the heart. Even sitting in your chair, practicing the breathing routines in this chapter, can make a positive impact on your cardiovascular health.

Chapter **4**

Adding Meditation to Chair Yoga

raditional Yoga teachings have always recognized the importance of meditation, and Western science has finally jumped on the bandwagon. More and more clinical studies have emerged over the years that recognize the advantages of adding meditation to your fitness or self-care regimen.

In addition to some of the overall benefits of Yoga, including things like stress reduction, managing chronic pain, slowing down your breath rate, and lowering your blood pressure, meditation may also

» Enhance your emotional well-being

» Increase self-awareness (both mentally and physically)

» Improve memory function

The list of potential benefits is just too significant to be ignored. This chapter makes the case for adding meditation to your regular self-care efforts. And, more than that, mediation can fit quite easily into your Chair Yoga routine.

Eyeing Meditation as a Core Component in Yoga

From a Yoga perspective, practicing meditation is easily as important as doing poses. Most traditions even recognize meditation to be an essential ingredient.

Claiming the power of your mind

Yoga therapists know that the mind can be both a cause of physical distress and a tool in resolving problems. Sometimes what's lurking in the subconscious mind manifests itself in ways that are challenging and even detrimental.

Meditation is a way to explore the mind, even beneath the surface, but it requires practice — and sometimes a little bit of bravery — to accomplish.

Considering common types of meditation

You can explore many types of meditation. Any one particular approach isn't necessarily the type that's right for you, so try a few techniques to see whether something resonates. The more common types of meditation include the following:

>> **Guided meditation:** In this style of mediation, you listen to the voice of someone leading the session (live or previously recorded), possibly talking about a specific theme (like gratitude or nature). The voice gives your mind something on which to focus. Some great meditation apps that include guided meditations are available.

>> **Breath-focused:** Sitting comfortably in your chair may be the perfect place to practice some breathing techniques *(pranayama)* or maybe just let your mind focus on simple inhales and exhales.

>> **Instinctive Meditation (IM):** Developed by meditation expert Dr. Lorin Roche, *Instinctive Meditation* believes that your body already knows how to meditate: "It's part of our built-in healing abilities." IM says you just need to find what works for you.

>> **Mindfulness:** Although mindful meditation may originate in the Buddhist tradition, it's probably one of the most popular types of meditation in the West. It's an approach that focuses on awareness — of your own thoughts and emotions. It asks you to observe without making assessments.

>> **Loving/kindness:** At first, this approach may seem more like an overly sentimental greeting card. But a growing body of Western clinical studies

suggest that it's actually a very powerful form meditation. You basically express feelings of love, forgiveness, and goodwill to the people in your life, including both friends and strangers and enemies.

>> **Visualization:** Using your own imagination to create an internal reality is a technique different forms of meditation use.

At a minimum, the idea is to mentally create a peaceful place or a happy idea, imagine how each of your senses would be stimulated in that reality, and ultimately let that positive energy soothe and strengthen your mind and body. In some disciplines, practitioners believe that what you visualize on the inside may manifest itself in the outside world.

>> **Prayer or spiritual meditation:** Simply put, this type of meditation strives for a connection with the divine. Most major religions, including Christianity, Judaism, Buddhism, Islam, and Hinduism, have strong traditions relating spiritual meditation. For anyone who doesn't seek the divine, this meditation can be a process of self-study or self-awareness.

>> **Moving meditation:** The process of coordinating movements with breath focuses the mind on the movement itself rather than the grocery list. Maybe, in some sort of cosmic irony, movement is a way to achieve focus, and even a stillness, of sorts (a stillness of purpose).

Yoga, even Chair Yoga, often strives to make movements or transitions from one posture to the next a moving meditation, but it's really an essential part of practices like Tai Chi and Qigong.

>> **Transcendental Meditation (TM):** The late Maharishi Mahesh Yogi popularized this technique back in the '60s, although its roots are in ancient Indian tradition. Typically using a *mantra* (a phrase or sound constantly repeated aloud or mentally), the practitioner attempts to clear their mind and find a sense of ease.

Meditating with the chakras

Simply put, a *chakra* (pronounced chalk-ra) refers to a primary location in the body where your life energy or spiritual power resides. Using the chakras in meditation is a common approach, especially in visualization.

REMEMBER

Chakras represent a much more sophisticated concept than these few paragraphs may imply. The good news is that the most dominant chakra model contains only seven chakras (see Figure 4-1), although many more actually exist:

1. **Crown chakra (sahasrara):** Found near the top of the head, the crown chakra represents a higher state of consciousness. Color: violet or white.

2. **Third eye chakra (ajna):** The third eye chakra sits in the middle of your forehead and is connected to your intuition or imagination. Color: blue or purple.

3. **Throat chakra (vishuddha):** Positioned at the throat, this chakra is connected to communication or self-expression. Color: blue.

4. **Heart chakra (anahata):** The heart chakra, found at the center of your chest, is related to your ability to love and to find joy. Color: green.

5. **Solar plexus chakra (manipura):** Located near belly button, the solar plexus chakra is primarily connected to self-confidence. Color: yellow.

6. **Sacral chakra (svadhisthana):** The sacral chakra, which is in your pelvic region, connects to sexuality as well as well-being. Color: orange.

7. **Root chakra (muladhara):** Positioned at the base of your spine, this chakra connects to your sense of stability or feeling grounded. Color: red.

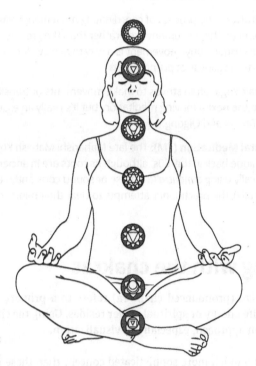

FIGURE 4-1:
Seven chakras.

Seeking Enlightenment Right from Your Chair

Meditators frequently sit cross-legged on the floor, often on a cushion (called a *zafu*). But many Yogic traditions encourage the use of a chair during meditation. You can visit your local meditation center or places like the Self-Realization Fellowship and see people doing just that.

The bottom line is that you want to minimize the distractions around you when you try to go inward and connect more with your mind, and the biggest distraction can easily be the discomfort from sitting cross-legged on the floor.

For many, sitting in a chair is more comfortable than sitting on the floor. If you're one of those people, Chair Yoga may support your efforts to meditate better than any other style of Yoga. Of course, if you *aren't* one of those people, feel free to take whatever position works for you.

TIP

Because you can actually do a Chair Yoga practice in a very limited space, it's a great way to practice meditation at work or while traveling. Whether you're sitting at your desk or perhaps on an airplane, train, or bus, you can close your eyes, tune out the world around you, and turn your thoughts inward.

Seeing How Meditation Slows Dementia

A growing body of research in Western medicine points toward meditation as an effective part of an intervention plan for dementia. Studies from places like Harvard show that a regular mediation routine can result in positive structural changes in the brain.

Anecdotal evidence from centuries-old Yoga tradition, as well as our own experience working with all kinds of people over the years, suggest that meditating truly does have a positive impact on people's ability to think and remember.

REMEMBER

Meditation is certainly not a cure for dementia, but it does seem to reduce symptoms in the areas of thinking problems and memory loss. And if you start a routine before you have symptoms, who knows; you may prevent or at least delay the onset of cognitive diseases like dementia.

As we discuss earlier in the chapter, meditation can ease stress and anxiety, which can contribute to dementia. Moreover, you may also be increasing blood flow to the brain, bringing in more oxygen and more fuel.

The free flow of *prana* (life force or energy) through your body is what Yoga believes keeps you healthy. One Yoga concept says, "Where your thoughts go, prana flows." Maybe allowing your focus to look inward does indeed increase the flow of prana through your brain and ultimately your body.

Decreasing Stress and Increasing Your Sense of Well-Being with Meditation

Some people tend to worry more than others. Age doesn't seem to matter; it's more about personality. In extreme cases, however, that worry or anxiety can lead to depression, which can have more serious consequences.

Whenever you experience a stressful situation, your body tries to help. Often, that help comes in the form of hormones that crank up your metabolism and get you ready to either run away from danger or stay and fight it. These hormones are adrenaline and cortisol. Both chemicals assist you in your fight-or-flight response by

>> Increasing your heart rate

>> Raising your blood pressure

>> Surging your energy

>> Raising your blood sugar levels

Of course, most of the time you don't want to trigger this fight-or-flight response. Meditation can help keep you relaxed and keep these stress hormones properly balanced (they don't go away).

REMEMBER

Chair Yoga itself helps you lower your stress and anxiety. Adding a meditation component to the practice only amplifies the results. If meditation truly can reduce that anxiety, maybe even help you sleep better, then you'll ultimately be more satisfied with life. That sense of satisfaction can have a profound effect on your physical health and your mental outlook.

Spending a Few Moments Meditating

We make this point earlier in the chapter, but it's worth saying again here: You can meditate a vast number of ways, and no one way is right for everybody. You need to try different approaches and see what you like. If you enjoy the experience, you're more likely to come back to it, and persistence is definitely the key.

As you try the following exercises on for size, start with the breath-focused meditation. You already know how to breathe; you've been doing it a long time on your own. The only thing you must do now is think about it — and start inhaling and exhaling just through your nose if that works for you. Head to Chapter 3 for more on the concept of nose breathing.

Breath awareness meditation

While the process of simply breathing is too often automatic, something we don't even think about, our bodies are very aware of just how important a lung full of fresh air can be. If you doubt that, deprive your lungs of air, and see how long you can hold out. Breathing is an essential part of life.

The following steps help you breathe with more awareness:

1. **Sit in your chair and get comfortable.**

   You can rest your back against the back of the chair, cross your legs, or put blocks or cushions underneath your feet. Though the focus here isn't about finding good posture, you may still want to sit tall so that your lungs and diaphragm can expand and move freely with each breath.

2. **Try to relax your whole body and remember to keep breathing — maybe in and out through your nose with your mouth lightly shut.**

   If you can't breathe solely through your nose, by all means use your mouth.

3. **Start to become aware of the pattern of your breath.**

   Where do you feel like the air is going? Into your chest? Into your stomach? Somewhere else?

4. **With your mind, follow your breath in and out, letting your breath rate slow over time.**

5. **Maintain this focus for a total of five to ten minutes.**

   If your mind starts to focus on other things, gently bring it back, knowing as you do that your mind is designed to move and explore. You can celebrate this capacity and still try to control it.

Meditation using visualization (Example 1)

Visualizing during meditation often involves an external voice leading you to a place of safety, of comfort, of pure sensual pleasure. In this exercise, you allow your own imagination to transport you to such a place, and then embrace the feelings of contentment and comfort that emerge within you.

1. **Sit in your chair and get comfortable.**

2. **If it feels okay, close your eyes and try to slow your breathing.**

   If it feels too unstable with your eyes closed, just stare down at the floor.

3. **Start to imagine that you're sitting somewhere in nature, maybe by a river or the ocean or in a deep forest.**

4. **Imagine what would touch your senses.**

   Can you hear the waves breaking or birds chirping? Can you smell the dense forest growth or the salty sea air? Maybe you even feel the warmth of summer day or the coolness of the evening.

5. **Gently breathe as you mentally explore the world you created in your mind.**

   It's the original virtual reality.

6. **Start to bring yourself back slowly.**

   Take time to appreciate this refuge you created, a place only you can go to, a place you can return to at any time.

Meditation using visualization (Example 2)

If, in the previous exercise, you let your mind take you to a beautiful place in nature, this exercise brings you upward, maybe into the sky, maybe into outer space. See where your imagination takes you and try to engage your senses along the way.

1. **Get comfortable in your chair.**

2. **If it feels okay, close your eyes and try to slow your breathing through your nose.**

   If it feels too unstable with your eyes closed, just stare down at the floor.

3. As you inhale, visualize that you feel lighter.

4. As you exhale, visualize that you start to float upward.

5. Continue this visualization, imagining yourself to be lighter and lighter, floating higher and higher.

6. Maintain this focus for about five to ten minutes.

WHERE DOES THE MUSIC COME FROM?

We sometimes struggle in Yoga to reconcile traditional Eastern thought with our more modern Western sensibilities. That challenge emerges when considering if music has a place in a meditation or Chair Yoga practice.

Like so many things, there's not a one-size-fits-all answer to this question. Most traditions acknowledge the healing power of sound, accepting prayerful chants or repeating mantras as part of a meditative journey. Still, that's a far cry from playing some contemporary ballad in the background while attempting to still your mind.

The fact is probably most meditation traditions frown on the use of music — playing tunes while meditating is highly discouraged. In our culture, however, music is a common accompaniment for most contemporary fitness activities. So, what should you do?

The answer, on one level at least, is simple: it's your practice, and you can do what works. There's plenty of Western science to support the idea that music can help to reduce stress or help you relax. So, if that's your meditation goal, maybe a pair of earbuds is going to be part of your essential equipment.

It is possible, however, that you want the internal journey of meditation to do more than just help you to relax. In that case, music could be a big distraction, especially if you choose the wrong song.

Ultimately, you can decide what you want to accomplish in the time you set aside for meditation and take complete comfort in knowing that whatever works best for you is absolutely the right choice.

2
Chair Yoga for the Body

Explore how Chair Yoga can target specific areas of the body from your neck down to your feet.

Check out the most-popular standing poses that use the chair, and decide whether this optional category of Chair Yoga is right for you.

Chapter **5**

Relieving That Pain in Your Neck

Neck pain is a pretty common problem, but addressing that pain can be tricky. The issue may be from muscles, joints, or nerves in this area, known as the *cervical spine*. The cause of the pain may be job-related, or perhaps from an injury, a sport, or some other hobby. Of course, certain types of neck pain are solely related to stress or anxiety.

Regardless of the cause, neck pain is all too real. Chair Yoga frequently focuses on the neck, not only to help alleviate that pain but to also avoid future occurrences of it entirely.

Banishing the Stress That Builds Up in Your Neck

Eliminating the causes of stress-related pain can be a problem in itself. Some stressors — work, family members, your commute, your nosy neighbor — are things you may have to learn to live with because they're unlikely to just disappear.

So if removing the cause isn't realistic (at least for now), your only alternative is to see whether you can decrease your stress response. Chair Yoga does just that by offering some targeted stretches and movements that may help loosen up those tight neck muscles that are fueling the discomfort. (We cover some of those later in the chapter.)

Feeling the effects of mental and emotional stress

Stress can be involved in a multitude of illnesses, including back pain and migraine headaches. But the neck and shoulders are the most common sites of tension in "the Western being."

Chair Yoga does two very important things for this problem:

>> Increases awareness of clenching patterns

>> Relaxes tight muscles

REMEMBER

If you can harness these Chair Yoga benefits, you put them in your self-care tool kit and hopefully find a way to ease stress-related pain and discomfort — especially in your neck.

Talking about text neck

Text neck is a popular term that refers to the pain you feel in your neck when spending too much time bent over a cellphone as illustrated in Figure 5-1. However, phones aren't the only culprits; neck pain or tightness can impact anyone who keeps their head tilted forward for prolonged periods of time (whether they're reading, knitting, or whatever). The point is, holding your head in some type of forward position can strain the muscles and ligaments in your neck, as well as stress the top of your spine (your cervical spine). Unfortunately, in contemporary society, electronic devices are the biggest culprits.

TIP

Whether you're 18 or 80, good posture is essential.

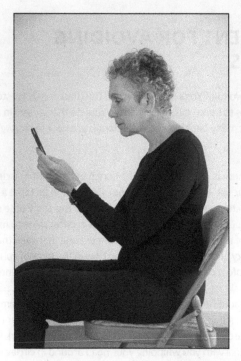

FIGURE 5-1:
Holding your
head forward
can lead to
"text neck."

Doing Chair Yoga for the Neck

Exercises that focus on the neck involve the top of your spine (your cervical spine), so a few guidelines are important.

WARNING

Many healthcare professionals warn against doing full head or neck rolls for a number of reasons (discussed in the nearby sidebar). Not only can you move your neck into unnatural positions, but you also risk compressing certain nerves or arteries. As always, check with your doctor if you think you have issues with your neck.

The good news is that Chair Yoga offers a number of neck routines that are generally considered safe. Here are a few you can try.

AN ARGUMENT FOR AVOIDING NECK ROLLS

Not all debates in the world of Yoga involve Eastern tradition versus Western science. A good example relates to head rolls — a common routine that we see in many different disciplines but that many health care professionals are now saying we should stop doing entirely.

The issue is that your neck is not only made of a bunch of different muscles, but it also contains the top of your spine (your cervical spine). Despite the fact that a head roll is a relatively basic move, tilting your head backwards while at the same time rotating it can sometimes force the neck into positions that cause the cervical spine to move well outside its normal range of motion — right into the danger zone. Between the risk of spinal injury and the possibility of compressing the blood flow in the back of your neck, some medical and fitness professionals believe it's best to just avoid this routine entirely.

When this book talks about holding your head too far forward, it's not simply because it looks bad (even though it does). It has more to do with the fact that your head is heavy, probably somewhere around 11 pounds. Your cervical spine has to work to support that weight, let alone deal with you whipping your head around in circles or maybe holding it backward for an extended period of time.

There are other great ways to stretch the muscles in your neck (some are described right in this chapter), but the latest clinical research says neck rolls are just not one of them.

Chin swings

This routine is basically a variation on a neck circle. Although stretching the neck muscles may be beneficial, doing a complete head circle can endanger the cervical spine (basically, the bones in your neck). Many medical professionals advise against the movement for just that reason.

In this routine, you limit the rotation of your cervical spine but still stretch some of the primary neck muscles.

1. **Sit upright, being mindful of your posture (see Figure 5-2).**

    Your hands can rest on your legs.

2. **Tilt your head down, bringing your chin close to your chest, but keep it comfortable (see Figure 5-3).**

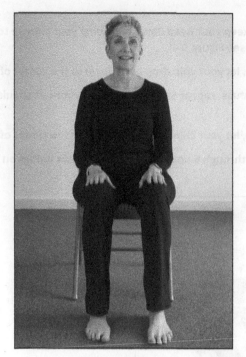

FIGURE 5-2:
Sitting with an upright posture.

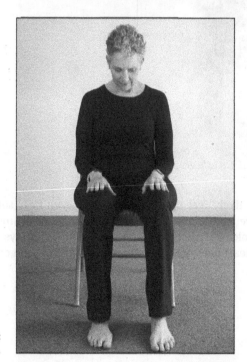

FIGURE 5-3:
Chin to chest.

3. As you inhale, keep your head down but swing your chin up toward your right shoulder (see Figure 5-4).

4. On your exhale, let your chin drop back down to the center of your chest.

5. On your next inhale, repeat Step 3 but toward your left shoulder (see Figure 5-5).

6. On your exhale, let your chin drop back down to the center of your chest.

7. Repeat Steps 3 through 6 until you've done six chin swings on each side.

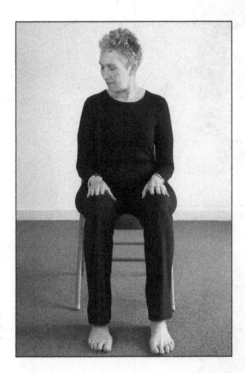

FIGURE 5-4:
Swinging your
chin toward your
right shoulder.

REMEMBER

Your neck will very likely feel tight, and you may even hear some cracking or popping as you move from one side to the other. But as with any movements or postures in this book, you shouldn't feel pain. Pain is always a sign to stop completely — or at least back off on the intensity until the pain disappears.

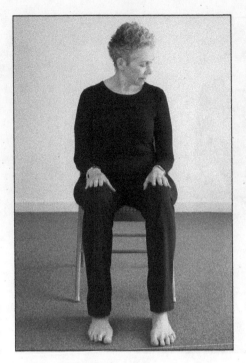

Neck range-of-motion stretch: Forward tilt

The next three routines are designed to stretch specific muscles in your neck. As always, don't work through pain; be ready to back off if necessary. Only move your head as far as it wants to go. So, for example, if you can't bring your chin all the way to your chest, only bring it as far as it wants to go. Your only goal here is to stretch out already tight muscles or to keep loose muscles from tightening.

1. **Sit upright, as tall as you can.**

   Your hands can rest on your legs, and your feet should rest comfortably on the floor (or on blocks, a stack of blankets, or some other prop that brings the floor up to your feet).

2. **On an exhale, tilt your head down, bringing your chin gently to your chest (see Figure 5-6).**

3. **As you inhale, bring your chin back up to the starting position in Step 1.**

4. **Repeat Steps 2 and 3 two more times, moving with your breath, and then hold your chin down for six seconds.**

5. **As you inhale, bring your chin back up.**

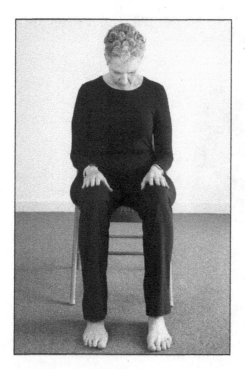

FIGURE 5-6:
Chin to chest
stretches the
back of the neck.

Neck range-of-motion stretch: Rotations

This routine stretches a new set of neck muscles — the ones that move your head like you're saying "no." The thing to concentrate on here is not letting your chin dip downward when you rotate.

1. Sitting tall in your chair with your chin level, take a big inhale.

2. As you exhale, rotate your head to the right, keeping your chin level (see Figure 5-7).

3. As you inhale, rotate your chin back to the starting position in Step 1.

4. Repeat Steps 2 and 3 two more times on the same side, moving with your breath, and then hold your rotation for six seconds.

5. On your next inhale, rotate your chin to the starting position.

6. Repeat Steps 1 through 5, rotating your head to the left.

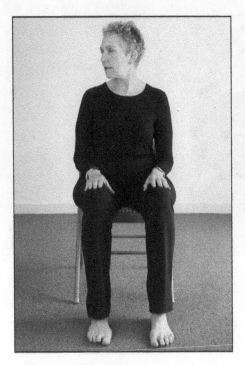

FIGURE 5-7:
Rotating
your head.

Neck range-of-motion stretch: Lateral head tilts

The last set of muscles being targeted here focus on the sides of the neck. Again, as you tilt, keep your chin up. Don't worry about your range of motion in any of these movements. Do only what you can, and you will probably find that you're able to stretch further as time goes on.

1. **Sitting comfortably but maintaining a good posture, take in a big inhale.**

2. **As you exhale, tilt your head to the right (see Figure 5-8).**

   Try not to tilt your head so that your chin drops toward your chest. You may notice a tendency to lean your whole body in the direction of the tilt. Try to keep your sitz bones (the bottom part of your pelvis that you're probably sitting on) pressed equally into the seat of your chair.

3. **As you inhale, tilt your head back to the starting position in Step 1.**

4. **Repeat Steps 2 and 3 two more times on the same side, moving with your breath, and then hold your third tilt for six seconds.**

5. **On your next inhale, tilt your head back up to the starting position.**

6. **Repeat Steps 1 through 4, tilting your head to the left.**

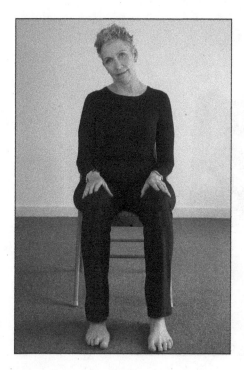

FIGURE 5-8:
Tilting your head
to the side.

Mirror on the hand

Intro text here: This routine is taken directly from *Prime of Life Yoga* (see Chapter 15) and adapted to the chair. It's a great way to stretch out the neck and shoulders.

1. Sitting comfortably but maintaining a good posture, place your hands palms-down on your thighs.

2. As you inhale, raise the back of your right hand to eye level (see Figure 5-9).

3. On your exhale, bring your right palm to the opposite shoulder and follow it with your eyes, bringing your chin down (see Figure 5-10).

4. As you inhale, bring your hand back in front of your face, keeping your eye on it as you bring it around to the right as much as is comfortable like in Figure 5-11.

5. On your exhale, lower your right palm back down to your right thigh.

6. Repeat Steps 2 through 5 five more times.

7. Repeat Steps 2 through 6 on your other side.

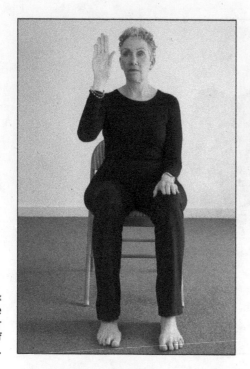

FIGURE 5-9:
Gazing at the
imaginary mirror
on the back of
your hand.

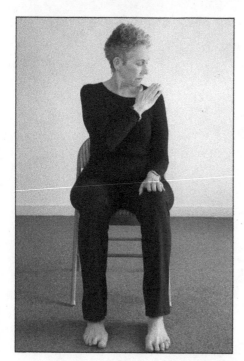

FIGURE 5-10:
Watching your
hand move to
your shoulder.

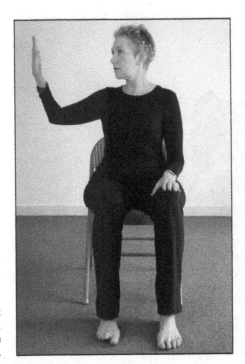

FIGURE 5-11:
Reaching out,
with your eyes on
the mirror.

Chapter **6**

Stretching and Straightening the Shoulders

The shoulders have a lot of poetic significance — they can carry the weight of the world, take on an criticism and responsibility, and even offer others a place to cry.

From a strictly anatomical point of view, though, the shoulders are complex structures made up of so many muscles, bones, and ligaments that keeping them all straight is hard. They're the primary ball-and-socket joints that let your arms move freely up and out in all directions.

There's an undeniable relationship between your shoulders and emotion, so you want to not only keep them physically in tune but also avoid making them the home for stress.

Looking at Where Tension Likes to Live

Stress is a common aspect of life that can impact people in different ways and to different degrees. If you increase the amount of emotional or physical stress in your life, your body may respond by doing any or all of the following:

>> Increasing your heart rate

>> Raising your blood pressure

>> Speeding up your breathing

>> Producing stress hormones like adrenaline

>> Tightening or tensing your muscles

All these things are fight-or-flight responses to stress, ways in which your body thinks it may be helping. And if you happen to need to stay and fight or to race away, some of these responses may make a lot of sense.

REMEMBER

The shoulders are often prime targets for the "tighter muscles" category. In fact, chronic shoulder pain caused by too much stress seems to be an all-too-common human condition.

Resisting the Tendency to Round

The first thing to think about when considering rounded shoulders is that it's just not a good look. Rounding your shoulders utterly compromises your posture, and you lose the fit look of having a strong spine.

But more than just aesthetics, your body may also experience additional stress trying to compensate for your new posture. For example, consistently holding your head too far forward adds extra weight (about the same as a bowling ball) that your body has to support.

REMEMBER

The good news is that you can easily fix a lot of bad habits, including shoulder rounding, if you put some thought into it.

Counteracting the Western lifestyle

Unfortunately, the lifestyle of many people in the West encourages shoulder rounding. Even the most routine activities can be responsible:

>> Hovering over a smartphone

>> Typing on a computer keyboard or laptop

>> Extended sitting, whether in a chair or car

>> Putting on makeup or shaving

>> Sitting on a toilet

>> Doing the dishes

>> Riding a bike

WARNING

Even the most beneficial activities can have some negative repercussions if you fail to maintain good form.

Improving your posture by channeling mom: "Sit up straight!"

As it turns out, Mom was right — about a lot of things, but especially that old chestnut "sit up straight!" Sitting erect demands good posture, and this book repeatedly talks about the health benefits related to having a good posture.

Poor posture can cause certain types of shoulder conditions, like *shoulder impingements* (an irritation of the rotator cuff) or shoulder rounding. If you make an effort to improve your posture now, you may head off these problems, and improve your overall flexibility in the process.

Of course, if you're currently feeling any type of shoulder pain, you should talk to your doctor.

Avoiding sitting too much

Science is still studying the negative effects of too much sitting, but enough red flags are already waving to warn about the seriously negative consequences of this seemingly harmless activity. Here, the problem is stiff or tight shoulder muscles.

REMEMBER

Your shoulders are particularly impacted when the extended sitting is behind your desk, maybe slumped over a computer or a stack of papers. When you're sitting with good posture, at an ergonomically correct desk, your posture is similar to your Yoga starting posture pose.

Surveying Chair Yoga for Your Shoulders

Your shoulders may not be the first thing you scrutinize when you're standing in front of a mirror, but strong, flexible shoulder muscles and well-lubricated joints keep your shoulders functioning properly. The following sections offer a few Chair Yoga exercises to help with that goal.

Shoulder shrugs: Part 1

Shoulder shrugs may seem like an overly basic routine, but they're a very effective way to build some awareness of your shoulders and upper back. The way to make these moves truly Yogic is to move with your breath as we discuss in Chapter 3. If you're breathing slowly, you're going to move slowly.

1. **Sit upright in your chair with your ears over your shoulders and your shoulders over your hips.**

   Be sure your shoulders are back (not drooping forward); sit naturally.

2. **As you inhale, raise both shoulders toward your ears.**

3. **As you exhale, let your shoulders roll back and then fall down (see Figure 6-1), returning to the starting position in Step 1.**

4. **Repeat Steps 2 and 3 five more times, moving with your breath.**

Shoulder shrugs: Part 2

Because your shoulders are ball-and-socket joints, moving them in all directions is important. This movement attempts to do just that.

1. **Sit upright in your chair with your ears over your shoulders.**

2. **As you inhale, raise both shoulders toward your ears.**

3. **As you exhale, let your shoulders fall forward toward your chest (see Figure 6-2) and return to your starting position.**

4. **Repeat Steps 2 and 3 five more times, moving with your breath.**

Shoulder shrugs: Part 3

Like so many Chair Yoga movements, this exercise may seem quite basic, but moving just one shoulder while keeping the other motionless can really be challenging.

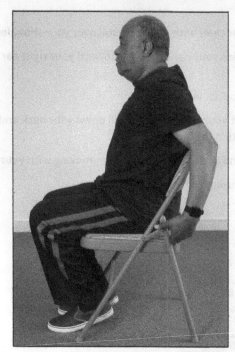

FIGURE 6-1:
Shoulders fall
backward.

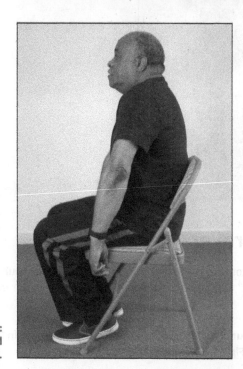

FIGURE 6-2:
Shoulders fall
forward.

1. Sit upright in your chair with your ears still over your shoulders.

2. As you inhale, raise your right shoulder toward your right ear (see Figure 6-3).

   Leave your left shoulder in place.

3. As you exhale, let your right shoulder fall down your back and return to the starting position in Step 1.

4. Repeat Steps 2 and 3 with the left shoulder, moving with your breath.

5. Repeat Steps 2 through 4 five more times.

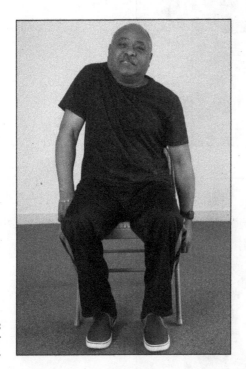

FIGURE 6-3:
Single shoulder shrug.

Wing and prayer

Not only does this routine work the muscles and joints in your shoulders and neck, but the "wing" movement also opens up (stretches) the muscles in your upper chest.

1. Sit upright in your chair with your hands in prayer position in front of your chest (see Figure 6-4).

2. As you inhale, take your bent arms out wide (see Figure 6-5).

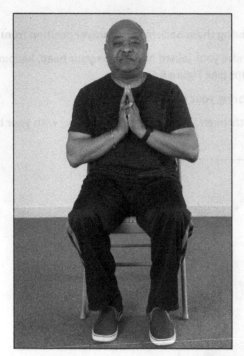

FIGURE 6-4:
Starting position.

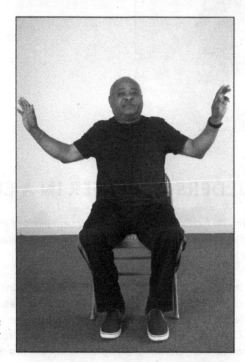

FIGURE 6-5:
Spreading your
wings.

3. As you exhale, bring them back into the prayer position from Step 1.

4. As you inhale, raise your joined hands over your head, keeping your eyes on your fingertips (see Figure 6-6).

5. As you exhale, bring your arms back down.

6. Repeat Steps 2 through 5 five more times, moving with your breath.

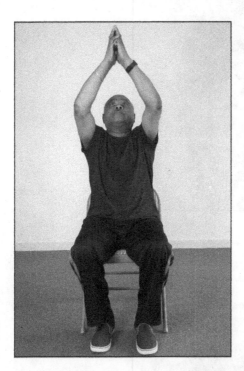

FIGURE 6-6:
Raising your
hands.

YOUR SHOULDERS ARE SAFER IN A CHAIR

While Yoga Therapists readily use Yoga principles to address all kinds of shoulder problems, the fact remains that too many shoulder injuries initially occur in traditional Yoga classes — but not Chair Yoga.

Of course, there are multiple reasons why these types of injuries occur in the first place: perhaps practitioners are ignoring warning signals from their own bodies. Maybe they're trying to compete with the people around them or with the hyper-mobile Yoga instructor in the front of the room. The biggest challenge, however, has to do with the simple fact that your shoulders are just not designed to support the sustained full weight of your body. All too often, Yoga asks your shoulders to do just that, but again, not Chair Yoga.

Consider how much stronger your hips are (your pelvis). By comparison to your shoulders, the hips are a much larger, much more durable structure, able to easily support your body weight (which, in fact, they are exactly intended to do). Your shoulders girdle, on the other hand, is a much smaller, more delicate configuration that's definitely challenged by doing even simple poses that shift your body weight onto your shoulders.

For the most part, Chair Yoga just doesn't do that.

Chapter **7**

Bringing Your Back
to the Forefront

alking about your back is a bit like talking about the United States of
America. Lumping together 50 different states with very different cultures
and people can be, at best, imprecise.

Similarly, "the back" is really an overall physical region that is actually comprised
of some very distinct components. You may already be aware of some:

» Top of the spine (base of the skull)

» Neck

» Back of the shoulders

» Shoulder blades (scapula)

» Traps (trapezius muscles)

» Lats (latissimus dorsi)

» Deep muscles of the hips and pelvis

» The spine as a whole

» The individual vertebrae of the spine

That's a lot of parts to keep flexible, moving, or strong. And it's not always easy. Back pain is one of the most common reasons people miss work, second only to the common cold. In fact, 80 percent of the U.S. population experience back pain at one time or another during their lifetime.

Doing what you can to keep your back healthy is very much up to you. Luckily, it's also a primary goal of Chair Yoga.

Supporting Your Spine with Yoga

An old saying in the Yoga world correlates the suppleness of the spine to fitness or youthfulness. People with a fit spine — those who demonstrate both good posture and flexibility — do indeed seem more physically fit. Yoga can offer you postures, movements, and even breath work that help keep the spine healthy and flexible.

TIP

Chair Yoga can improve your

>> Stress level and related tight muscles (particularly in the upper part of your back)

>> Overall posture

>> Muscle tone and strength (think about all of the muscles in your back that help support your spine)

REMEMBER

Of course, Yoga can also lead to back problems if you try to push things too far. The secret is to pay attention to how any movement or pose makes you feel and avoid anything that resembles pain or even discomfort.

You may be pushed by the people around us or your own egos. But doing what's good for your body rather than what's good for your ego or sense of competition is the key to making Yoga work for you.

Remembering to work your upper back

Roughly speaking, your *upper back* includes your neck and shoulders. Any of the following may be the cause of pain or tension in that area:

>> Anxiety and stress

>> Overworking the muscles

> » Bad posture (often simply due to bad habit)
>
> » Injury

REMEMBER

Your shoulder muscles also reach up your neck and to the bottom of your skull. If those muscles get tight, that tension may even cause headaches.

Touching on your lower back

The *lower back* more or less starts somewhere just below your rib cage and ends somewhere around your pelvis. This portion of your back is sometimes referred to as the *lumbar region*. One of the primary jobs of the muscles here is to support your spine.

Although the lumbar spine is durable, it's the part of your spine that supports most of your body weight and can lead to problems. Common causes of low back pain can include

» Lifting something heavy

» Inactivity

» Fear, anger, and stress

» Twisting the spine (such as while playing sports or lifting something heavy)

» Falling down

» Poor posture

» Underlying spinal conditions like lumbar strain/sprain, disc issues, joint issues due to inflammation or disintegration, *stenosis* (narrowing of the spinal canal), and arthritis

Keeping the muscles strong and flexible and the joints mobile and lubricated helps you avoid many of these problems. That's where Chair Yoga can come in.

Breaking Down Chair Yoga for the Back

As we note earlier in the chapter, the back covers a lot of muscles. For the most part, the routines in the following sections target different areas.

WARNING

If any movement causes you pain or discomfort, don't do it; talk to your health care provider. The cause may be rather benign, and an expert can help you over-come any discomfort or recommend you avoid certain movements and poses altogether.

Alternating arm raises in a chair

Raising your arms over your head uses back muscles that need to be stretched and strengthened as well as engages your shoulder joints.

1. **Sit upright in your chair with your hands resting comfortably on your thighs.**

2. **On an inhale, raise your right arm toward the ceiling and rotate your head to the left (see Figure 7-1).**

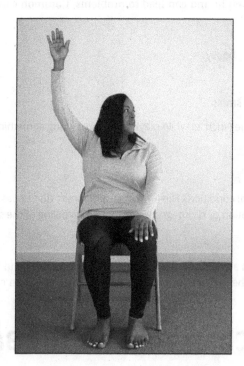

FIGURE 7-1:
Raising your
right arm.

3. Lower your arm as you exhale and turn your head back to the center.

4. On your next inhale, raise your left arm toward the ceiling and rotate your head to the right (see Figure 7-2).

5. On an exhale, lower your arm back down and turn your head back to the center.

6. Repeat Steps 1 through 5 for a total of five times.

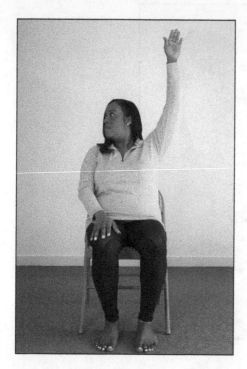

FIGURE 7-2:
Raising your
left arm.

Seated cat/cow

The cat/cow routine is a great way to warm up your spine — especially if you happen to be independently moving each one of the 24 vertebrae that make up your spinal column. Chair Yoga offers the perfect version of this classic movement.

1. Sit upright in your chair with your hands resting comfortably on your thighs.

2. **As you inhale, slide your hands up toward your hips and bring your elbows back, arch your back, and allow your head to tilt slightly backward (see Figure 7-3).**

   This position is the cow pose part of the exercise. Keep your elbows close to your rib cage as you move them. You don't need to let your head fall too far back.

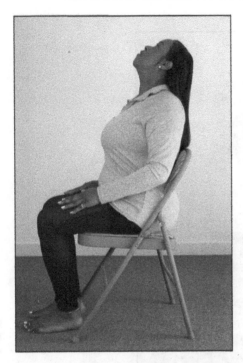

FIGURE 7-3:
Cow pose in
a chair.

3. **As you exhale, slide your hands back toward your knees, round your back like a Halloween cat, and allow your head to tilt slightly forward (see Figure 7-4).**

   Now you're in the cat pose.

4. **Repeat Steps 1 through 3 nine times.**

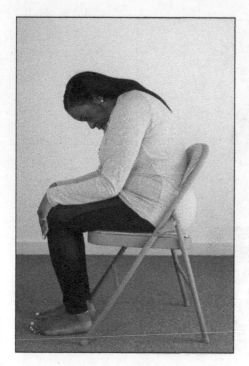

FIGURE 7-4:
Cat pose in
a chair.

Seated side bends

Among other areas of the body, this movement targets your lower back muscles
that can suffer from too much sitting or immobility.

1. Sit upright in your chair.

2. On an inhale, grab the side of your chair with your left hand and raise
    your right arm toward the ceiling (see Figure 7-5).

3. As you exhale, bend sideways to the left and bring your right hand over
    your head in the same direction (see Figure 7-6).

    You may feel yourself tipping sideways. Try to bring yourself back down into
    the chair so that you're sitting with even pressure on both sides.

4. Hold the side bend for about six breaths.

5. On your next inhalation, return to your upright position and then release
    both arms so that you're in the starting position from Step 1.

6. Repeat Steps 1 through 4 on the other side.

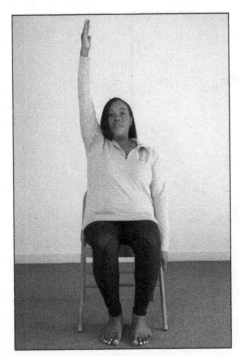

FIGURE 7-5:
Getting ready
to bend.

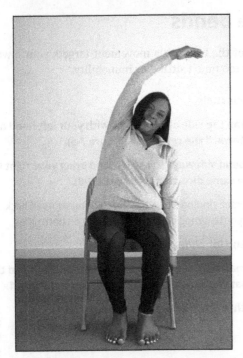

FIGURE 7-6:
Bending to
the left.

Seated camel

This pose requires more of a *static* (nonmoving) hold, but it opens the chest in the same way the cow pose does in the earlier "Seated cat/cow" section. This posture is a great one for stretching out the front of the body, from your chest down through your thighs. It's particularly helpful in compensating for all the rounding of the spine that occurs so frequently in the course of a day (including hunching over a keyboard or cellphone, driving, and even cooking).

1. **Sit upright in your chair, lengthening your spine by allowing the top of your head to rise toward the ceiling.**

2. **As you inhale, reach behind you with both hands and grab the chair, perhaps slightly tilting your head backward and looking up toward the ceiling (see Figure 7-7).**

WARNING

   Don't tilt your head back too far. Many physical therapists and chiropractors advise against doing so because of all the nerves near the back of the neck. Just slightly raising your chin and your eyes is enough.

3. **Hold this pose for six to eight breaths.**

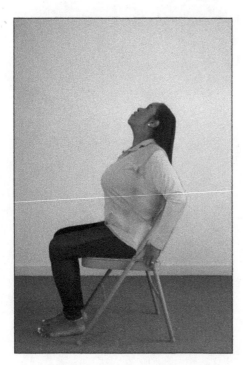

FIGURE 7-7:
Seated camel
pose.

ALL ABOUT THAT BACK MOVEMENT

Sometimes, even the most routine movements — bending forward or leaning back, for example — can appear to be the cause of pain. Yet these movements are also very essential as you go about your day, and you don't want to permanently give them up.

While this sidebar in no way attempts to replace the critical assessment made by your doctor or other health care professional, it's probably safe to say that immobility is not going to alleviate your problem — and will probably make it worse. You may need to stretch and strengthen your muscles, including your core, if you want to alleviate back pain. But, again, only when the doctor says you're ready to start that kind of work. And you may even need some professional advice to help you determine the best exercise routines in your rehabilitation.

Of course, there's always the risk of over-working your back, so that's why it makes sense to get some professional guidance. But doing nothing — especially not moving — will only make things worse. And who knows? Maybe Chair Yoga will be just what the doctor orders.

Chapter **8**

Paying Attention to Your Abdominals

Aside from looking good in your swimsuit, well-toned abdominal and core muscles are important for other, more practical reasons:

» Aid your body's movements

» Support your back

» Help you stand tall

Whether you're doing things for fun, like swimming and golfing, or doing things you have to do, like pushing a vacuum cleaner or a lawnmower, strong abdominals and core muscles bolster your efforts all along the way.

Supporting Your Back from the Front: Creating a Strong Core

As with the back (see Chapter 7), don't think of your core as a single muscle. It's really composed of a group of muscles:

>> Back muscles

>> Abdominal muscles

>> Certain hip muscles

>> Respiratory diaphragm and pelvic floor

The following sections introduce some of the benefits of a strong core.

Avoiding back pain

Health care professionals who regularly see patients for back pain often attribute part of the problem to weak abdominals or core muscles. As Yoga therapists, we certainly see exactly that. One of the reasons weak core muscles can cause back problems is that certain back muscles are forced to compensate. Your spine takes over the job that other core muscles are supposed to do.

Unfortunately, that compensation can lead to back strain or injury, especially if the body moves in some unusual way that otherwise would've been prevented if the core and abdominals were strong.

Obviously, the best way to avoid these kinds of back problems is to keep your abdominals and core strong. We give you ways to do that in the later section "Adding Chair Yoga for the Abdominals and Core."

Helping your posture

The abdominals and core play an important role in keeping your spine stable and aligned. If those muscles are weak, your posture and overall stability suffer.

Bad posture makes you look older and less fit than you really are (see Figure 8-1).

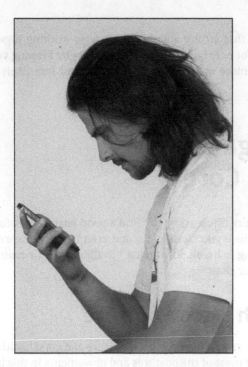

FIGURE 8-1:
Bad posture.

TIP

Good posture not only makes you look more physically fit but also

>> Helps keep you stable and balanced

>> Gives your lungs more room to expand and your diaphragm more room to move

>> Protects your back

Contributing to better balance

So, you know from the discussion earlier in this section that your core is made up of more than just your abdominals. And although your core isn't the only factor in maintaining your balance, it's definitely an important one. A strong core helps keep you stable and standing tall, and prevents additional strain on other parts of your body that may otherwise struggle to compensate for a lack of balance. Simply put, your core supports your spine.

Many Chair Yoga routines focus on this part of your body. Before you begin any of these routines, it may be beneficial to bring your attention to the various parts of your core. Maybe even tighten your abdominal muscles, as if the person next to you was about to send an elbow into your solar plexus. That simple contraction may actually enhance the work you are going to do.

REMEMBER

The bottom line is that strong abdominal muscles working together with other parts of your core not only help your overall posture by keeping you more upright but also keep you more stable, better balanced, and less likely to fall and get injured.

Adding Chair Yoga for the Abdominals and Core

In a Yoga class, you're often asked to "find a good posture." Before jumping into chair routines that help you stretch-out and even build your core and abdominal muscles, we're going to break down what "finding a good posture" means when you're sitting in your chair.

Sitting with a good posture

We discuss the relationship between good posture and good health throughout the book, and the fact is most of the postures and movements in this book require you to first sit up tall. Here's what we mean by that:

1. **Sit upright in your chair, with your ears over your shoulders.**

2. **Allow your head to float upward, as if the top of your skull were being magnetically drawn toward the ceiling.**

3. **Slide forward in your seat and place your feet flat on the ground.**

   Even if your feet reach the ground, sliding forward creates some needed space behind you.

   As we discuss in Chapter 2, don't dangle your feet. If your particular stature or the height of your chair prevent your feet from naturally touching the floor, you can put something under your feet.

4. **Mentally "feel" your posture.**

   Notice how your core and abdominal muscles help you sit upright.

You can see what good posture in a seated position looks like by checking out Figure 8-2.

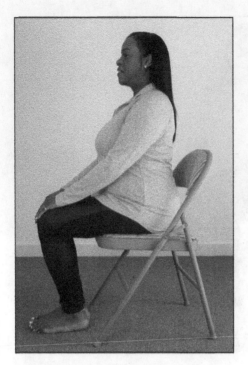

FIGURE 8-2:
Sitting with
good posture.

Bent knee lifts

These knee lifts engage your abdominals as well as stretch your thighs.

1. **Sit upright in your chair.**

2. **Take a big inhale and then raise your right knee as you exhale (see Figure 8-3).**

   Note: You don't have to grip the sides of your chair as you lift (as the model does in Figure 8-3), but you can do so if it helps.

3. **As you inhale, lower your knee back down until your foot returns to the ground.**

4. **On your exhale, raise your left knee.**

5. **On your inhale, lower your knee back down until your foot returns to the floor.**

6. **Repeat Steps 2 through 5 five times.**

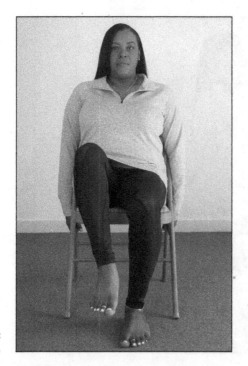

FIGURE 8-3:
Lift your knee.

Seated boat pose

Boat pose is a traditional Yoga posture, and this Chair Yoga version offers virtually the same benefits.

1. **Sit upright in your chair, sliding forward a bit (leaving space behind you).**

2. **Grip the sides of your chair with both hands.**

3. **Raise both knees and lean back.**

    Note: You can do this step with one leg at a time if that makes more sense for you. In that case, you complete the exercise with that leg and then repeat it with the other.

4. **Try to straighten your leg (as shown in Figure 8-4a) or legs (as shown in Figure 8-4b), but don't worry if you can't.**

5. **Make sure you aren't holding your breath and hold the pose for two to four breaths.**

6. **Lower your leg or legs.**

7. **If you raised only one leg in Step 3, repeat Steps 3 through 6 with the other leg.**

    Of course, if you did both legs, you can also repeat the exercise.

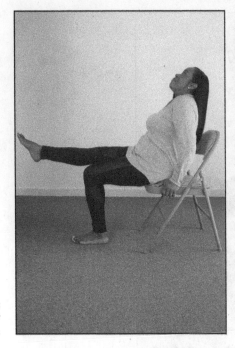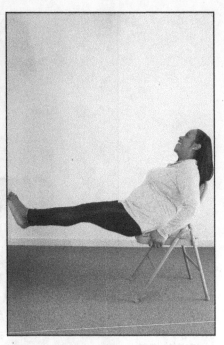

FIGURE 8-4:
Straighten your
raised leg(s).

TIP

For an added challenge, raise your hands from the sides of the chair and extend your arms straight forward after you've lifted your knee(s) in Step 3. But if you feel your posture being compromised, you're feeling pain, or you notice you're holding your breath, you may want to continue gripping the chair for support.

Seated twists

In Yoga, twisting poses are thought to have a long list of benefits. Chair Yoga offers various versions of a twist, including this one that focuses on your abdominals. Notice how it engages the muscles around your waist.

1. Sit upright in your chair with your hands on your thighs.

2. As you inhale, rest your right hand on your left knee and reach for the back of the chair with your left hand (see Figure 8-5).

3. On your exhale, twist your entire torso toward the back of the chair, still sitting tall (see Figure 8-6).

4. Hold the pose for five more breaths.

    This is a torso twist; resist the urge to twist with your neck.

REMEMBER

5. Release the twist on an exhale, bringing your body back around to the starting position in Step 1.

6. Repeat Steps 1 through 5, twisting in the opposite direction.

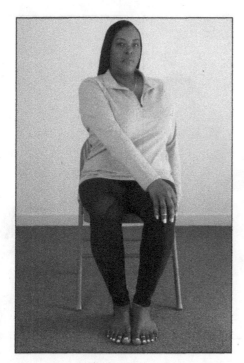

FIGURE 8-5:
Bringing your
right hand to
your left knee.

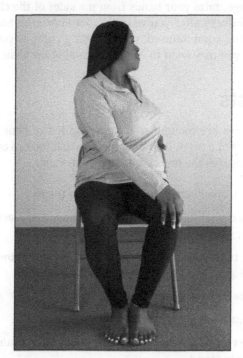

FIGURE 8-6:
Twisting your
torso.

Extended side angle

This pose actually targets a number of muscles, but it certainly works the side of your waist — specifically, your obliques.

1. Sit upright and swing your right leg over to the right side of your chair.

2. Keep the rest of your torso facing the front and straighten your left leg out to the left (or simply sit with your knees wide).

3. As you inhale, bring your straight arms up into a *T*-shape (or if you're having an issue extending both arms, just extend your right arm like in Figure 8-7), still facing the front of the chair.

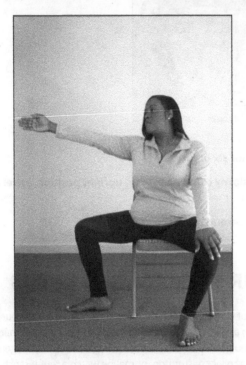

FIGURE 8-7:
Preparing for
extended side
angle pose.

4. As you exhale, bend your right elbow and let it rest on your right thigh with your palm up.

5. On an inhalation, bring your straight left arm up, over your left ear, and let your palm face outward.

6. Exhale and let your gaze move up underneath your raised arm (see Figure 8-8).

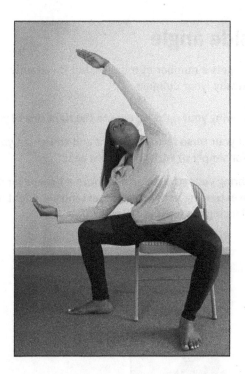

FIGURE 8-8:
Extended side
angle pose in
a chair.

7. Hold this pose for six breaths.

8. On an exhale, slowly come back to an upright position, lowering your arm back down.

9. Repeat Steps 1 through 8 on the other side.

WHEN YOUR STOMACH'S IN KNOTS

There's a definite line of communication between your stomach and your head. That link is often referred to as the "gut-brain connection." You experience that connection firsthand every time you get "butterflies" before giving a presentation, get "sick to your stomach" anticipating a roller coaster ride, or maybe watch a "gut-wrenching" old movie.

If such a link does indeed exist, consider how what's going on in your head can affect your stomach — even your digestion. Cramps, acid reflux, and indigestion can all stem from a stressful drive to work or telephone conversation with an annoying relative.

Once you acknowledge that stress or anxiety can indeed play a part in any number of stomach ailments, it then becomes readily apparent how stress-reducing activities like Chair Yoga (including breath work and meditation) can help to help relieve or even prevent those ailments.

Chapter 9

The Hips Don't Lie

I f you happen to be a professional hula dancer or an Elvis impersonator, chances are you can skip this chapter. Your hips may already be getting plenty of movement and strengthening.

For most people, however, the more they sit (on the couch, behind the wheel, or at a desk), the tighter and even weaker their hip muscles seem to become. This degeneration can create a host of problems involving a lot more than just the hips.

In the Yoga tradition, hips are often thought to be a vessel of sorts for emotions or tension brought on by day-to-day living or by some traumatic event. The simple movements in Chair Yoga are thought to release some of that tension.

Of course, some Western medicine practitioners don't endorse this belief, but even Western doctors recognize the impact that too much stress can have on the body. Everyone can agree that healthy, mobile hips are good for lots of reasons.

Taking Care of Your Hips

The hips are complex structures involving various muscle groups, including the *abductors* (muscles that rotate the leg or move it away from the body, out to the side), the *adductors* (which move your leg toward the center of your body), the extensors, and the hip flexors. The hips are also big ball-and-socket joints that have a direct impact on other parts of your body, like your lower back and knees. The best way to keep any of your joints healthy is to keep them moving — stretch them a little to allow them to maintain their normal range-of-motion.

Belly dancers know the benefits derived from a simple shimmy:

>> Lubricates the hip joints

>> Strengthens supporting muscles

>> Eases back tension

>> Improves posture

REMEMBER

The goal of Chair Yoga is to achieve all these benefits, and the movements and routines in this book help you do just that.

Knowing what it means to open your hips

In Yoga, *opening your hips* means stretching or lengthening certain muscles that are part of or close to the hip. These muscles can get tight, and the joints themselves can get stiff. You can wind up with not only sore hips but also a sore back or sore knees.

Opening and closing your hips may produce the very health benefits we describe earlier in the chapter. This action simply moves all those hip muscles and keeps them strong and flexible.

TIP

In Chair Yoga, you can easily tell when your hips are open. Notice in Figure 9-1a, both hips are initially facing forward (closed position). In Figure 9-1b, the right leg is then swung open (almost like an open gate). When you know the difference between the two positions, you can feel whether your hips are opened or closed.

Preventing injuries by strengthening your hips

REMEMBER

Your hips can be prone to injury if you try to push them too far or too intensely. Pay attention to how any movement or posture feels, and don't tolerate pain or discomfort.

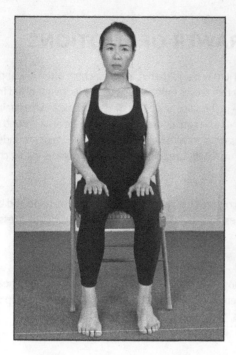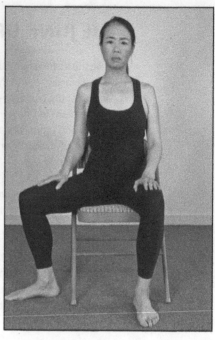

FIGURE 9-1:
Opening your
hips.

Strong, flexible hips help prevent certain types of injuries. Even the simple act of walking depends on healthy hips.

WARNING

If your hips are too weak, you may experience

>> Chronic leg pain

>> Knee pain

>> Back pain

>> Foot pain (even plantar fasciitis)

In addition, strong hips help you with balance and stability and thus prevent injuries relating to falls. If you want to keep moving, having healthy, flexible hips offers a multitude of health benefits.

THE JUNK DRAWER OF EMOTIONS

While the science behind it may be quite thin, Yoga teachers often talk about the hips being a place in our body that stores emotion. Perhaps this idea evolved from the concept of the chakras — in this case, probably the root chakra (we explain the chakras in more detail in Chapter 4). The root chakra is located in the area around the pelvis and the hips and is typically associated with helping you feel secure or grounded. Perhaps the ideas of insecurity or instability are associated with problems in that chakra or that area of the body.

Even Western science recognizes the relationship between the mind and body. It often attributes physical manifestations of pain or disease with feelings of stress, depression, or anxiety.

Regardless of the cause — either from some emotional crisis or perhaps simply from sitting in one place for too long — tight hips can be the enemy to good health. It just makes sense to move them and even stretch them with some kind of hip opening routine. Enter Chair Yoga.

Getting a Handle on Chair Yoga for Hips

The thing about having tight hip muscles, as discussed earlier in this chapter, is that it may not only cause pain in your pelvic area but also in your low back. The following Chair Yoga routines target your hips, stretching and strengthening those often-overlooked hip muscles that tend to become overly tight — especially from immobility.

Hip circles

This simple movement can help stretch and strengthen the muscles around the pelvis. Feel free to reach down with each hand and hold on to the sides of your chair if doing so helps you feel more grounded in your chair.

1. **Sit in your chair toward the front edge of your seat to help to ensure that your feet are flat on the ground.**

   If your feet don't naturally touch, you can use a prop to lift the ground as we describe in Chapter 2. Be sure you leave space between your back and the back of the chair (see Figure 9-2).

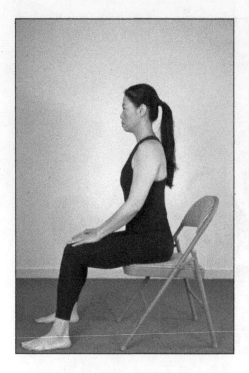

FIGURE 9-2:
Sitting tall with
your feet on
the ground.

2. **Lean forward a bit (hinging from the hips) and start circling your upper torso, breathing in as you circle back and breathing out as you circle forward (see Figure 9-3).**

   Even though this is a continuous movement, a slow enough tempo allows you to move with your breath.

3. **Keep circling with this breathing pattern for five more breaths.**

4. **Reverse the direction of your circle, still breathing in the same way.**

5. **Keep circling with this breathing pattern for five more breaths.**

You're welcome to close your eyes during this routine if you feel comfortable and stable.

Seated pigeon

Pigeon pose is a great way to open up your hips, but many Yoga teachers see the posture as too advanced. In the chair version shown here, you're going to get all the benefits of a deep hip stretch while staying safe.

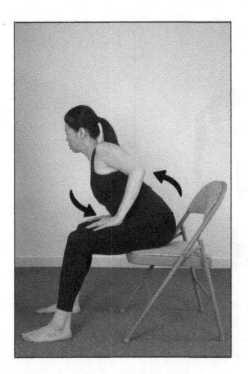

FIGURE 9-3:
Hip circles.

REMEMBER

Of course, the best way to avoid injury is to listen to your body. If this hurts, just don't do it.

1. **Sit upright in your chair with your feet on the ground or a prop.**

2. **Bring your right ankle onto your left knee (crossing your leg like in Figure 9-4) and lift your right toes toward your right shin.**

   If this position is painful for you or causes discomfort, again, just don't do this pose.

3. **Hold this cross-legged position for five breaths.**

4. **On an inhale, uncross your legs, and then exhale as you return to the starting position in Step 1.**

5. **Repeat Steps 2 through 4 on the other side.**

TIP

If you feel like you need a deeper stretch, assume the position in Step 2 and then sit tall as you inhale and lean forward on your exhale hinging from the hips (see Figure 9-5). Bending forward from the hips rather than rounding your spine increases the intensity of the stretch more quickly. *Remember:* This addition is an optional step. Don't do it if it hurts.

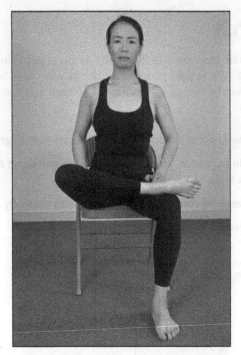

FIGURE 9-4:
Seated pigeon.

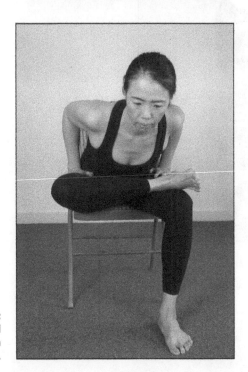

FIGURE 9-5:
Seated
pigeon with a
forward lean.

Seated march

Marching in your chair may seem a little silly at first, but think of how many muscles you're using. The longer you march, the heavier your legs are going to feel, and soon you may be struggling to lift your knees and maintain your easy breathing.

1. Sit upright in your chair with your hands resting on your thighs.

2. Begin to march in your seat, bringing one knee up and down and then the other (see Figure 9-6).

3. Continue this marching movement while breathing normally.

    When your breathing starts to become labored, you can stop.

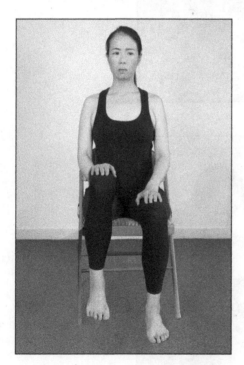

FIGURE 9-6: Marching in your chair.

Chapter **10**

Getting a Leg Up

Ballet dancers aren't the only ones who need to keep their legs in great shape. The daily demands you put on your legs are significant, but they're also so routine that you can easily forget about them when it's time to focus on your health. When you're walking down the aisle of a grocery store, you want your legs to help you stay upright and to propel you forward. They need to be strong. Unfortunately, because people tend to sit so much, leg muscles can be underused and grow weak.

We discuss how the entire chain works together to help your mobility in Chapter 12. The *lower chain* includes not only your feet and ankles but also your legs (plus knees), hips, and spine. Focusing on the legs during your Chair Yoga routine helps keep the chain strong and healthy.

This chapter focuses on your legs, specifically your

» Upper legs (the front of your thighs and your hamstrings directly in the back)

» Lower legs (your shins and calves)

» Knees

Checking out Your Legs

The front of your upper leg, your thigh, is also referred to as your *quadricep* or *quad*. (Now you can impress your friends if that ever comes up at a dinner party.) As you may be able to guess, this part of your leg is made up of four different muscles that work together.

The *hamstrings* are located at the top of the back thigh (just behind the quadricep), and that structure is made up of three muscles working together.

The quads and hamstrings help bend and straighten your leg. When one stretches or lengthens, the other gets shorter. One important thing to keep in mind here is that you want to keep them all at the same level of fitness or strength. An imbalance here can lead to a strain of the weaker muscles if asked to keep up.

Located on the back of your legs, just above your ankles, are your calf muscles. In addition to helping you stand and walk, these muscles also allow you to push off with your feet.

Your shins, on the other hand (well, leg), are located at the front of your lower legs, and they may feel more like a bone. The shinbone is actually the *tibia*. It probably supports more weight than any other part of the leg, and it anchors important muscles that keep you from tripping.

Knowing Knees Need TLC, Too

The knees are an important part of your legs and an essential structure in the chain we cover earlier in the chapter. They provide you with support and stability and allow you to stand upright and move.

REMEMBER

If you've had knee replacements (or any joint replacements, for that matter), talk to your health care provider before beginning Chair Yoga.

Staying aligned

Because the knee is basically just a hinge joint, it's designed to move in one direction, back and forth. If you try to move your knee sideways or twist it, you'll definitely feel some resistance — and maybe even sustain an injury.

You can avoid problems by keeping your knees properly aligned. That typically means your knees, whenever they bend and straighten, move in the direction your toes point (see Figure 10-1).

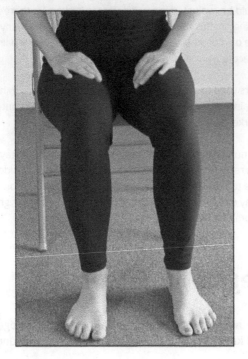

FIGURE 10-1:
Proper knee
alignment.

Encouraging free movement

TIP

The best thing you can do for your knees is to keep them moving. Doing so increases the production of *synovial fluid* (which basically functions like a lubricant and feeds your joint surfaces).

That's not to say that your knees can't wear out. All the joints in your body are subject to wear and tear over time, but keeping your joints moving and well lubricated may slow that wear and tear and keep you going.

Leg muscles support the knees

The thing to remember about your knees is that they include tendons, muscles, and ligaments. Although keeping them moving freely is important (see the preceding section), the surrounding leg muscles are what truly lend them support. If those muscles become weak, it may impact the stability of your knees.

CRAMPING YOUR STYLE

Leg cramps are an all-too-common problem. You may know just what it's like to spring out of bed in the middle of the night to walk off a cramp in your calf or thigh. Of course, regular cramping should be evaluated by your doctor to make sure there's not something more serious going on. But chances are you're just among the many people who experience the routine pain of an occasional leg cramp. And while the pain may be quite intense, the impact on your health is practically nonexistent.

Back in the day, doctors used to prescribe quinine-based medications to help with cramps. But the FDA raised some serious safety concerns, and drugs containing quinine were taken off the market.

Fortunately, there are non-pharmacological interventions. Aside from staying well hydrated — which can require finding a certain balance if you also consider how many trips you want to make to the bathroom at night — you need to keep your leg muscles well stretched. You may even want to consider some easy leg routines right before bed — maybe even from Chair Yoga.

Chair Yoga for Legs and Knees

Just because you're not standing doesn't meant that Chair Yoga isn't going to target your legs and knees. Each of the routines in this section does just that.

Seated warrior one pose

Warrior one is a good posture for many different reasons, but we include it in this chapter because of its leg and knee benefits.

1. **Sit upright in your chair with your knees facing to the right (see Figure 10-2).**

   Sitting toward the front edge of your chair may be helpful for this exercise, but be careful you don't become unstable.

2. **Bring your left leg back, making it as straight as you can.**

   If your left leg doesn't want to go back or straighten, bring it back only as far as it wants to go, or just open your legs.

3. **Extend one or both arms over your head (see Figure 10-3); you may choose to hold on to the chair with your right hand.**

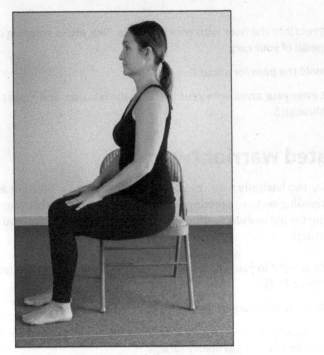

FIGURE 10-2:
Preparing for
seated warrior.

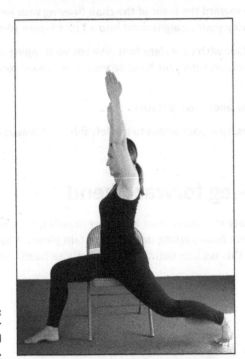

FIGURE 10-3:
Raising your
hands in seated
warrior one pose.

4. Press into the floor with your right foot (like you're stepping on the gas pedal of your car).

5. Hold the pose for about five breaths.

6. Lower your arms, spin your knees to the left side, and repeat Steps 1 through 5.

Seated warrior two pose

Warrior two basically requires you to find the same leg position as warrior one in the preceding section: pressing into the floor with the foot of your inside leg while opening the hip or even putting your other leg straight behind you (stretching that hamstring).

1. Sit upright in your chair with your knees facing to the right (see Figure 10-2).

2. Bring your left leg back, making it as straight as you can.

   If your left leg doesn't want to go back or straighten, bring it back only as far as it wants to go, or just open your legs.

3. Turn your torso toward the front of the chair (leaving your legs where they are) and bring your straight arms into a *T* (see Figure 10-4).

4. Press into the floor with your right foot (like you're stepping on the gas pedal of your car) and turn your head so your gaze is over your right hand (see Figure 10-4).

5. Hold the pose for about five breaths.

6. Lower your arms, spin your knees to the left side, and repeat Steps 1 through 5.

Seated one-leg forward bend

Some Yoga teachers say that more than any other muscles, tight hamstrings prevent Yoga practitioners from getting deep into certain poses. Whether this fact is or isn't true for you, this routine definitely targets those hamstrings.

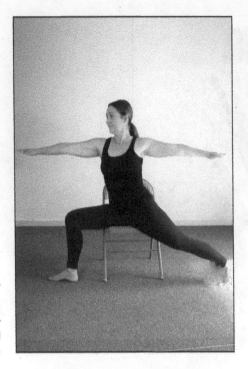

1. Sit upright in your chair with your hands on your thighs.

2. As you inhale, extend your right leg straight out with your heel on the floor.

3. On an exhale, slide both of your hands down your right leg toward your foot as you carefully bend forward (see Figure 10-5). Only go until you feel the stretch (no pain!).

   Your tight hamstring is probably what's going to prevent you from bending as far forward as you want to go. Don't try to compensate by forcing your back to bend further than it already is.

4. Hold this position for a total of six breaths.

5. Repeat Steps 1 through 4 on the other side.

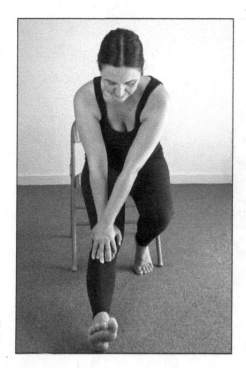

FIGURE 10-5:
Bending toward
your foot.

Chapter **11**

Arming Yourself

Although Yoga is definitely not a religion, many of the early Indian teachers who popularized the practice — even in the United States — were also devout Hindus.

As a result, many Hindu deities, like Lakshmi or Ganesha, are familiar figures to Hindus and Yogis alike. And if you look at art featuring these deities, you'll notice that many of them are shown with multiple arms. Indeed, Yoga — and therefore Chair Yoga — comes out of a tradition where arms represent superior power.

Even in our Western culture, we need strong arms to do a multitude of routine tasks. This chapter focuses on these all-important limbs — and not just getting them to look good.

Keeping Your Arms in Shape for Lifting, Reaching, and Hugging

Your arms allow you to reach out for things like cellphones, car keys, and even food. The arms connect on one end to the shoulders and on the other end to the hands. Like most structures of the body, your arms are made up of muscle, ligaments, and bone, all of which need to be maintained. The primary muscles of your arms are these:

>> Biceps

>> Triceps

>> Forearm muscles

The arms also involve multiple joints:

>> **Elbow:** A hinge joint connects your upper and lower arm and allows the arm to bend.

>> **Shoulder:** Your upper arm bone *(humerus)* fits into the socket. You can read more about shoulders in Chapter 6.

>> **Wrist:** Your lower arm bone *(radius)* fits into the socket. We cover wrists in Chapter 12.

Beautiful biceps

Your biceps help other, less well-known arm muscles with tasks like lifting. They support and stabilize the arms and surrounding structures, so keeping them toned is important.

TECHNICAL STUFF

Big bicep muscles were historically a sign of masculinity. Today, a well-toned bicep more likely indicates a certain level of physical fitness on people of any gender.

TIP

While Yoga can be a good way to build muscle, particularly when you're using your body weight as resistance, Chair Yoga tends to avoid that type of work (for any number of reasons). If you do want more focus on building muscle — maybe your biceps — take a closer look at Chapter 20. Adding a dumbbell or two to your routines (like in the bicep routine) helps to build muscle more quickly. The thing to keep in mind is that even light dumbbells will seem heavy if you do enough reptations. Just be sure that working with dumbbells (or any other type of added weight) is right for you.

Functional forearms

Your forearms work together with other arm muscles. They especially help the rotation of the arm itself, as well as the movement of the elbow, hands, and wrists.

REMEMBER

The concept of a chain or *kinetic chain* refers to how certain structures or muscles work together to achieve a certain goal. Strong forearms allow the other muscles in the chain to do their jobs.

Exceptional elbows

The elbow is where the upper arm bone (the humerus) meets the forearm bones (the radius and *ulna*). It's actually a hinge joint that primarily moves forward and backward (with very limited motion in other directions).

The elbow joint itself is basically held together by various ligaments and tendons, leaving the *ulnar nerve* somewhat exposed. You may know that nerve better by its other, usually inaccurate name, the funny bone.

Tennis elbow: Not just for tennis players

You've probably heard of tennis elbow, though the only thing you may know about it is that it's quite painful. *Tennis elbow* typically refers to the swelling of the tendons in the elbow.

Though tennis players and other athletes are certainly prone to this condition because of the repetitive arm motion of their sport, anyone who performs the same arm movements over and over is at risk to develop it.

Your doctor may suggest over-the-counter pain medications like aspirin (or the less inflammatory acetaminophen) along with rest to soothe the tendons. In more extreme cases, surgery may be required. Your doctor will guide you toward any potential remedies that are right for you.

Causes of elbow other problems

In addition to repetitive motion, other things can cause elbow problems such as stiffness:

>> Arthritis (typical joint problem)

>> Bursitis

>> Fractures

>> An injury (maybe from a fall)

>> Surgery of some kind

Of course, your healthcare professional can help you diagnose any problem you may be experiencing.

Though Chair Yoga isn't a treatment for these conditions, it does help keep the joint moving and maintain flexibility and good alignment.

Examining Chair Yoga for Arms and Elbows

So many postures and movements in Yoga seem too basic to be useful, but that isn't the case. Each of the routines in the following sections is easy enough to do and has huge potential benefits. Whether you're stretching tight muscles or moving joints that don't get enough movement, these arm and elbow routines can play a big role in keeping you strong and limber.

Elbow flex

Here's a very simple movement that targets the elbow joint. It's actually part of the Joint Freeing Series from India, brought to the West by Yoga therapy pioneer Mukunda Stiles.

1. **Sit upright in your chair with your arms straight out in front of you, your hands open, and your palms toward the ceiling (see Figure 11-1).**

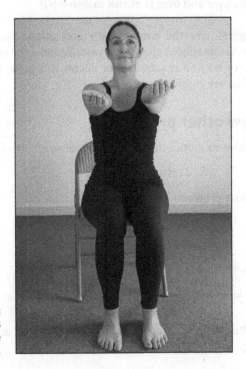

FIGURE 11-1:
Sitting with palms toward the ceiling.

2. **On an exhale, bend your elbows (keeping them at the same level) and bring your knuckles to your shoulders (see Figure 11-2).**

   If you can't actually bring your knuckles all the way back, go as far as you can without pain. Your range of motion will increase over time.

3. **Repeat Steps 1 and 2 five more times, moving with your breath.**

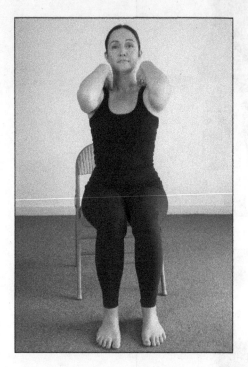

Forearm rotation

This is another gentle movement that (among other things) keeps your forearms limber.

1. **Sit upright in your chair with your arms straight out in front of you, your hands closed into fists, and your palms toward the ceiling (see Figure 11-3).**

2. **On an inhale, rotate your arms (keeping them at the same level) so that the palms of your closed hands now face the floor (see Figure 11-4).**

3. **Repeat Steps 1 and 2 five more times, moving with your breath.**

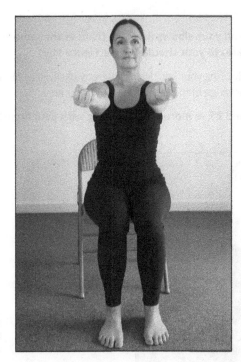

FIGURE 11-3:
Sitting with arms
straight out.

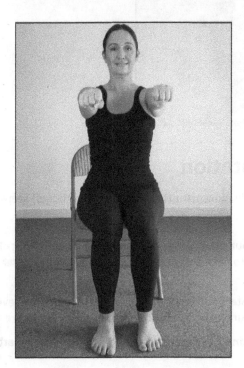

FIGURE 11-4:
Rotating
straight arms.

Newspaper

In the newspaper routine, your arms move in all directions. It also targets the upper body and can be a great way to bring some movement to the neck and shoulders (which we cover in Chapters 5 and 6, respectively).

1. Sit upright in your chair with your back long and your head floating up.

2. Inhale; as you exhale, move both hands up to eye level with your palms facing you as though you were looking at a newspaper (see Figure 11-5).

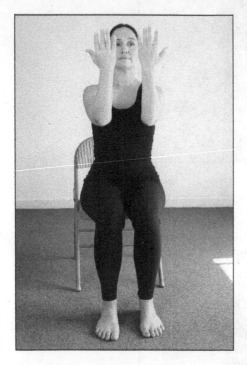

FIGURE 11-5: Looking at the newspaper.

3. As you inhale, lift both hands, following them with your eyes and head, until your hands are just above your forehead (see Figure 11-6).

   Try not to tilt your head too far back when you're looking up at your hands.

4. As you exhale, bring your chin down to your chest without moving your arms (see Figure 11-7).

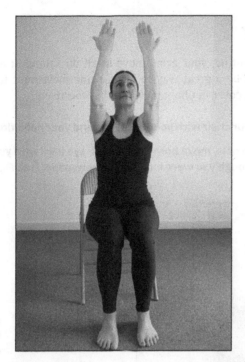

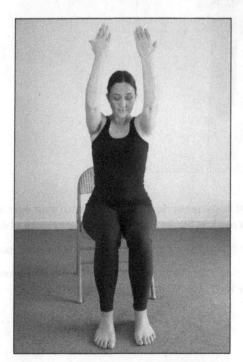

5. As you inhale, move your arms out to the sides like wings so your hands are at about shoulder height, lifting your chest and looking straight ahead (see Figure 11-8).

6. As you exhale, extend your bent arms forward like they're going over a log and round your back like a camel as you look down (see Figure 11-9).

7. As you inhale, lift your chest; rotate your elbows and palms inward as you raise your hands back to eye level just like in Step 2 (see Figure 11-10).

8. Repeat Steps 1 through 7 four to six times.

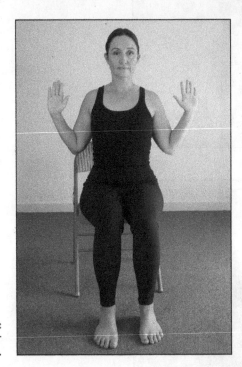

FIGURE 11-8:
Spreading your
wings.

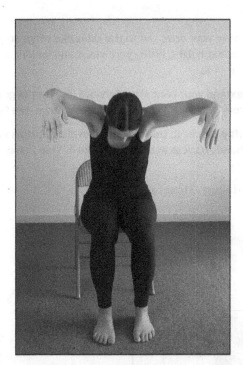

FIGURE 11-9:
Rounding.

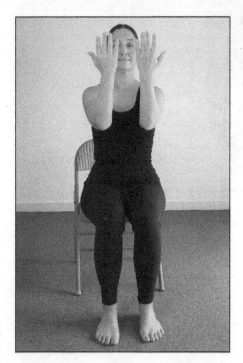

FIGURE 11-10:
Raising your
head again.

LOSING YOUR BAT WINGS

Over the years, the same question keeps coming up in class: "Can Yoga help me get rid of my arm flab?" The answer to that question is an unequivocal no — or yes. Or, it probably can, but only in conjunction with other efforts.

The issue is, in most cases (certainly not all), arm flab stems from too much fat on the arms. And as you probably already know, you can't "spot reduce" — you can't perform arm routines and expect to lose fat specifically on your arms.

These Chair Yoga arm routines will help to strengthen and tone your arms, but you also need to deal with the excess fat by doing some kind of cardio work. (Don't forget, despite what these power Yoga classes might tell you, your breath and heart rate should remain slow throughout your practice.) It also may be useful to talk to a dietician if your think bad eating habits could be working against you.

Still, these Chair Yoga routines can tone and strengthen your arms and help get them in shape for a sleeveless blouse or a tank top.

Chapter **12**

Ankles and Feet: Bearing All the Weight

The famous physicist Stephen Hawking once said, "Remember to look up at the stars and not down at your feet." But so much is happening down at your feet, and if you're dealing with foot or ankle pain, it may be the only place you're looking.

Strong ankles and feet are so important to your overall health and well-being. You can easily take for granted everything you ask them to do every day. From walking and running to standing in one spot or balancing, you obviously rely on those structures to keep you upright, stable, and moving. And they're certainly on the frontline in bearing your body weight. Chair Yoga offers some targeted routines that focus on all the related bones, joints, muscles, and ligaments that make up these critical parts of the body.

Understanding Why Foot and Ankle Health Are So Important

Strong, flexible feet and ankles allow you to move about freely and to stay safely upright.

The act of walking involves many areas of the body, but the feet are what hit the ground and then lift, and the ankles help them touch and lift off at just the right angle. Problems in the feet and ankles may lead to abnormalities in the way someone walks (their gait).

REMEMBER

Chair Yoga can help to keep the muscles of the feet and lower leg strong and flexible and the joints well lubricated.

Part of the kinetic chain gang

Your feet — which include your ankle joints — make up the first link in what's sometimes known as your body's kinetic chain. Without going into too much anatomy, the *kinetic chain* refers to the ways in which different parts of your body work together to allow for various types of movement. The chain typically includes the following structures; you can read more about them in the listed chapters:

>> Ankles

>> Knees (Chapter 10)

>> Hips (Chapter 9)

>> Lower, middle, and upper back (Chapter 7)

This linking means that the pain or discomfort you feel in one part of your body may have its source in another part. For example, your knee pain may actually be the result of a limited range of motion in your feet and ankles. Your knee is working too hard to compensate for what your ankle and foot should be doing.

Bones in the balance

Each foot has about 26 bones and over 30 joints. The ankles themselves are actually large joints composed of three more bones each. In total, that's . . . a lot of bones.

All these bones are susceptible to fractures and other bone-related maladies. Even *osteoporosis* (a serious decline in bone density) can lead to fractures in the foot.

WARNING

What makes things like fractures even more problematic is that the blood flow coming to this area of the body can be limited, making the healing process that much more sluggish.

Moving in the Right Direction with Chair Yoga for Ankles and Feet

Even in a Yoga practice, the feet and ankles may not get the attention they deserve. Fortunately, many of the movements and postures in a typical Yoga class, especially the standing postures, do stretch and strengthen the feet and ankles, even if it's more incidental than intentional.

The following Chair Yoga movements offer a very gentle but also very powerful approach to maintain healthy feet and ankles.

Flexing and extending your feet

Since your feet are made up of so many bones, muscles, ligaments, and tendons, there's a lot to keep in shape. Yet these complex structures, despite all what we ask them to do, are frequently ignored in many wellness routines. Not only will this simple routine help to stretch and lubricate your feet and ankles, it may also help to reduce foot cramps.

1. Sit upright in your chair with your feet on the ground.

2. Extend your right leg straight out in front of you (see Figure 12-1).

3. As you exhale, flex your foot back toward you with your toes together (see Figure 12-2).

4. On your inhale, point your foot (see Figure 12-3).

5. Repeat Steps 3 and 4 five more times, moving with your breath.

6. Repeat Steps 2 through 5 with the other leg and foot.

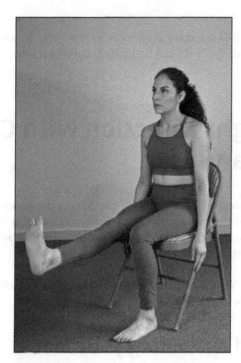

FIGURE 12-1:
Leg extended with a neutral foot.

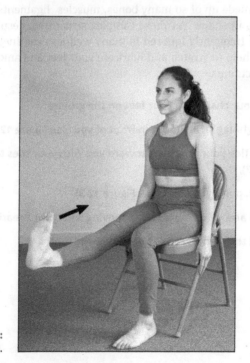

FIGURE 12-2:
Foot flexed.

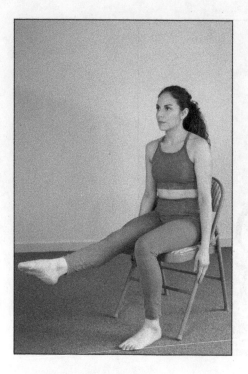

FIGURE 12-3:
Foot pointed.

Circling your ankles

Circling your ankles is a basic movement, but it's a great way to stretch the muscles in your feet and ankles. You may choose to do these stretches early in your routine to help warm up your muscles and prevent over-stretching.

1. Sit upright with a long back and your feet on the ground.

2. Extend your right leg straight out in front of you.

3. As you gently breathe, circle your ankle to the right (see Figure 12-4) for four breaths.

    Remember to breathe in and out through only your nose if possible.

4. Repeat Step 3, changing the circling direction to the left for a total of five breaths.

5. Lower your right foot back to the floor.

6. Repeat Steps 2-5 with the other leg and foot.

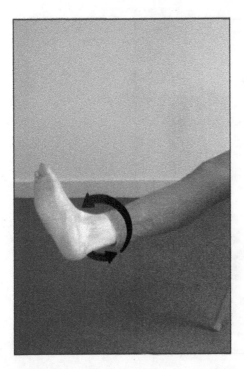

FIGURE 12-4:
Ankle circle.

Flexing and extending your toes

The toes are an important part of the foot. They help with balance and walking — and they deserve some real attention. This routine isolates the toes, again providing stretching of the muscles and maybe even strengthening.

1. Sit upright in your chair with your feet on the ground.

2. Extend your right leg straight out in front of you (see Figure 12-5).

3. As you inhale, spread your toes back toward you (see Figure 12-6).

4. On your exhale, scrunch your toes together (see Figure 12-7).

5. Repeat Steps 3 and 4 five more times, moving with your breath.

6. Repeat Steps 2 through 5 with the other leg and toes.

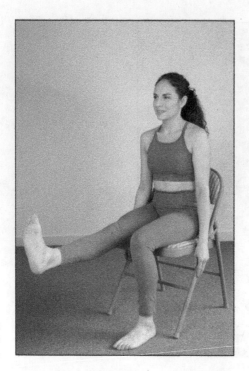

FIGURE 12-5:
Sitting with an
extended leg.

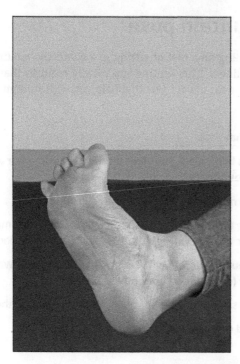

FIGURE 12-6:
Spread toes.

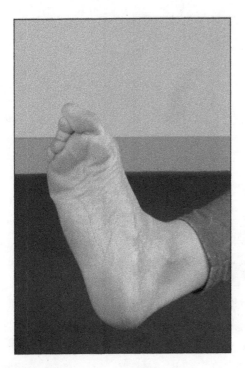

FIGURE 12-7:
Scrunched toes.

Seated mountain pose

Whether you're standing on a mat or sitting in a chair, the mountain pose is one of strength and sturdiness. This routine specifically requires that you pay attention to the anchoring areas of your feet that help you with standing and maintaining your balance.

1. **Sit tall in your chair.**

2. **With both knees bent, place your feet on the floor with your ankles directly below your knees.**

3. **On an exhale, firmly press your feet into the ground.**

   You should notice the feel of your big toe mound, your little toe mound, and the center of your heel (shown in Figure 12-8) pushing into the floor equally.

4. **Press down through your feet while even distributing your weight on the seat of the chair (don't allow your body to tip).**

   Make sure you're still sitting tall, with your head floating toward the ceiling.

5. **Continue to hold this position for six to eight breaths.**

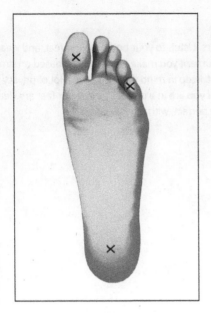

FIGURE 12-8:
Diagram of
pressure points
on the foot.

BAREFOOTIN'

While people have traditionally practiced Yoga in bare feet, that approach has certainly evolved over the years, especially as Yoga has become more "Westernized." There are now various types of "Yoga socks" available, some with toes, some without, some with a non-slip soles, some without. And they can, in fact, reduce how much you slip — or, if slipping isn't such a big issue (like it probably isn't in Chair Yoga), they can at least keep your feet warm on an otherwise cold floor.

Still, there may be some very good reasons to practice barefoot, and there may also be good reasons to wear Yoga socks — or even shoes.

Again, the deep-rooted Yoga tradition believes if you're barefooted, you're closer to the earth and to the earth's energy. More practically, it may be hard to do certain feet, ankle, or toe routines if your feet are bound in socks or shoes. Plus, basic anatomy tells us that our toes help us to balance, even walk. Maybe we can more effectively build the muscles in our feet by keeping them bare.

You may, however, be dealing with some kind of injury or medical condition that recommends additional support for the feet. Perhaps you have orthotics. Some podiatrists even say that doing Yoga in bare feet puts an unnatural strain on certain muscles and can lead to injury.

(continued)

(continued)

The decision is ultimately yours. Listen to your body, to your feet, and wear or don't wear what seems right. Of course, if you make your decision based on simply being self-conscious about bare feet, keep in mind that you have a lot of privacy when practicing Chair Yoga at home. And if you are in a public class, if your feet are clean and your toenails clipped, your feet are perfect, with or without shoes.

Chapter **13**

Don't Forget the Fingers, Hands, and Wrists

The hands and wrists typically work so closely together that thinking of them separately is difficult. Yet they're distinct structures that often have unique functionality and therefore require unique ways of keeping them healthy.

In this chapter, we review some of the activities that negatively impact your hands and wrists and give you some ideas about how to ease any pain you may be experiencing (or maybe even avoid that pain in the first place).

Preventing or Relieving Stiff Fingers and Hands and Painful Wrists

REMEMBER

The hands and wrists have almost 30 bones and about the same number of muscles.

Modern technology brings some risks to hand and wrist health. People spend an inordinate amount of time tapping on computer keyboards (or texting on miniature ones) and holding their phones to their faces.

These habits can lead to the *repetitive stress injuries* that sometimes happen when you do the same motion over and over. The best example is *carpal tunnel syndrome*, which occurs when swelling in this area puts pressure on the median nerve (we discuss that nerve further in the later section "Meditating on the median nerve"). It's common in people who spend a good portion of their day on a computer.

TIP

We provide some Chair Yoga exercises for counteracting hand, finger, and wrist strain later in the chapter, but here are a few other lifestyle adjustments that may help:

» **Take more breaks.** Holding your hands and wrists in the same position for an extended period of time may tighten them or even cause them pain.

   Note: A number of popular phone apps are available that remind you to take breaks at regular intervals.

» **Check your desk ergonomics.** *Ergonomics* refers to how items are designed and arranged for safe and efficient use. It's a very popular term because so much physical pain, including hand and wrist problems, stems from a person's spatial relationship with their computer. For example, the angle at which your fingers touch the keyboard can be critical.

» **Stretch.** A simple stretch has so many benefits for your hands and wrists. You may even be able to alleviate some pain.

Addressing arthritis attacks

Think of *arthritis* as a condition where the joints just wear out over time. Over time, and for many reasons, your joints can become worn. This wear and tear is a process that can begin early in life and lead to changes, including in your hands.

Chair Yoga offers a variety of benefits for relieving or even preventing arthritic pain:

» **Lubricates the joints:** Moving and stretching helps keep your hand joints (and all joints) lubricated. Immobility causes stiffness and pain, but the thoughtful movements in Chair Yoga may alleviate or prevent that pain.

» **Reduces stress:** Stress puts the body in a state of anxiety, in fight-or-flight mode, and that state can trigger an arthritis flare-up. Stress reduction, the kind associated with Chair Yoga, can have the opposite impact. A regular Chair Yoga practice could actually be part of your ongoing pain management strategy for dealing with arthritis pain.

Meditating on the median nerve

Several different nerves help control your arms, wrists, and hands, but the median nerve seems to be involved in some of the most common problems in this area of the body. The *median nerve*, shown in Figure 13-1, runs through the wrist up to the fingers.

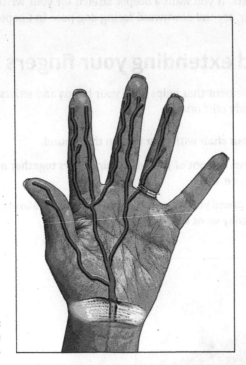

As we note earlier in the chapter, carpal tunnel syndrome is the result of pressure on the median nerve. This pressure can cause a tingling sensation — or even numbness — in your hand and wrist.

Choosing Chair Yoga for Fingers, Hands, and Wrists

The hands and wrists are critical parts of your anatomy that are easy to overlook — until something happens to them.

The lifestyle tips we outline in the earlier section "Preventing or Relieving Stiff Fingers and Hands and Painful Wrists" certainly apply to keeping your hands and wrist healthy, but Chair Yoga offers its own approach to target those areas, such as the exercises in the following sections.

Note: The routines we outline here provide safe and effective ways to stretch out your hands and wrists. If you want a deeper stretch for your wrists and can practice out of your chair, try the downward facing dog pose in Chapter 14.

Flexing and extending your fingers

Here's a simple movement that helps keep your hands and wrists from stiffening up and loosens already stiff ones.

1. Sit upright in your chair with your feet on the ground.

2. Extend both arms in front of you with your fingers together and pointed upward (see Figure 13-2).

3. As you inhale, spread your fingers as wide as you can, allowing them to curve a little if they want to (see Figure 13-3).

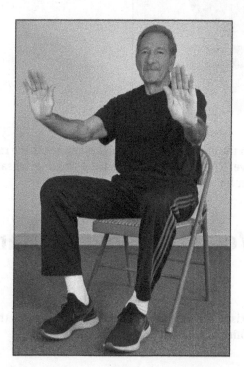

FIGURE 13-2: Arms extended with neutral hands.

4. On your exhale, squeeze your fingers into a tight fist (see Figure 13-4).

5. Repeat Steps 3 and 4 five more times, moving with your breath.

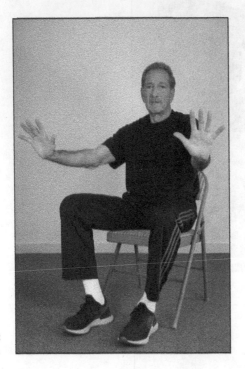

FIGURE 13-3:
Fingers spread.

Advanced finger exercise

If you deal with pain in your hands, stretching your muscles and moving the joints can help. While your doctor may prescribe a painkiller or even give you an injection, here's a routine you can try right in your chair.

1. Sit upright in your chair with your feet on the ground or a prop.

   Head to Chapter 2 for more on using props to make the ground higher.

2. Extend both arms in front of you parallel to the floor.

3. Turn your palms up (see Figure 13-5).

4. Place your thumbs at the tips of your index fingers on both hands (see Figure 13-6).

   Notice that you're doing the fingers on both hands at the same time.

5. Let your breath just flow through your nose slowly as you slide your thumbs to the base of your fingers and then back up.

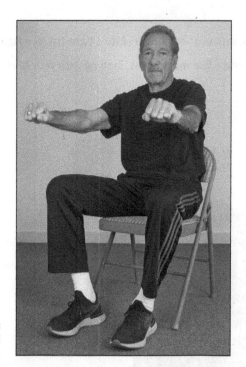

FIGURE 13-4:
Fingers closed
into fists.

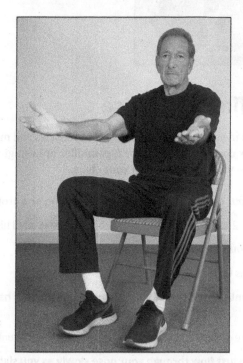

FIGURE 13-5:
Arms out and
palms up.

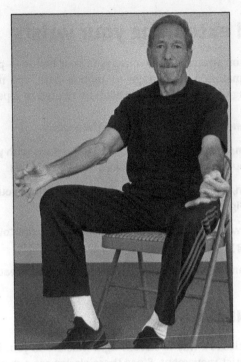

FIGURE 13-6:
Hands in starting position.

6. Before separating your thumb and finger, bring them into the position in Figure 13-7 and flick.

7. Repeat Steps 4 through 6 with your middle, ring, and little fingers (both hands at the same time).

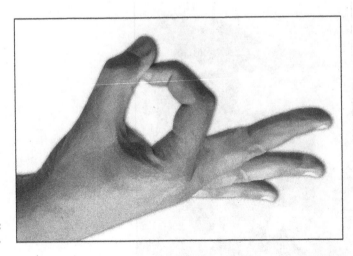

FIGURE 13-7:
Flick position.

Flexing and extending your wrists

This routine focuses on stretching the muscles in your hands — primarily around your wrists. If you maintain your range-of-motion here, you may reduce your chances of developing wrist problems, particularly related to repetitive motion.

1. Sit upright in your chair with your feet on the ground.

2. Extend both arms in front of you parallel to the ground with your fingers together and your palms facing downward (see Figure 13-8).

3. On an inhalation, point your fingers upward which brings your wrists into extension (see Figure 13-9).

4. As you exhale, swing your fingers downward so they point toward the ground, bringing your wrists into flexion (see Figure 13-10).

5. Repeat Steps 3 and 4 five more times, moving with your breath.

Circling your wrists

Performing wrist circles is a way to stretch tight muscles in your hands, focusing on another type of wrist movement. Since these circles are a good way to loosen up the wrists, it may make sense to do this early in your Chair Yoga routine.

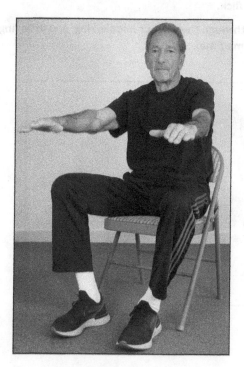

FIGURE 13-8:
Extended arms
with wrists
neutral.

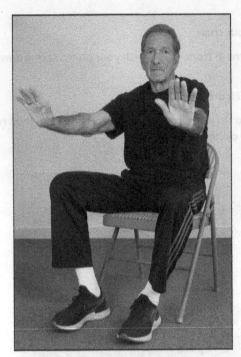

FIGURE 13-9:
Wrists in extension.

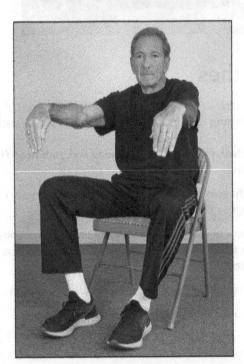

FIGURE 13-10:
Wrists in flexion.

1. Sit upright in your chair.

2. Extend both arms in front of you with your palms facing down (see Figure 13-11).

3. Make fists (see Figure 13-12).

4. Circle your hands in one direction about six times and then reverse the direction of the circles.

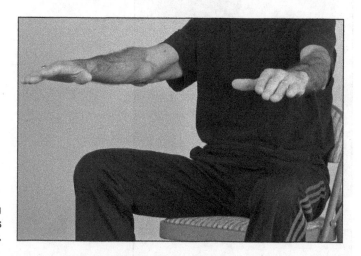

FIGURE 13-11
Extended arms with palms down.

Wrist stretches

The following wrist stretches appear in many different types of fitness training. What makes the following routine specifically Yogic is your breath.

1. Sit tall in your chair, keeping your back long and your head reaching toward the ceiling.

2. Extend your right arm in front of you with the palm of your hand facing outward (see Figure 13-13).

3. Use your left hand to pull your right fingers toward your body, giving your right wrist a nice stretch (see Figure 13-14); hold the stretch for about ten breaths.

   Make sure you aren't pulling so hard you cause pain or discomfort.

4. Repeat Steps 2 and 3 with your left wrist and right hand.

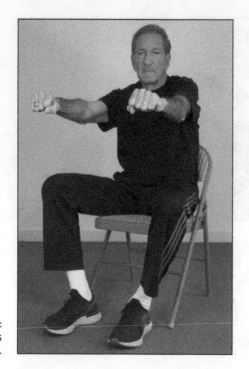

FIGURE 13-12:
Extended arms
with fists.

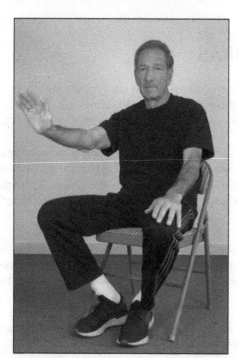

FIGURE 13-13:
Preparing for a
wrist stretch.

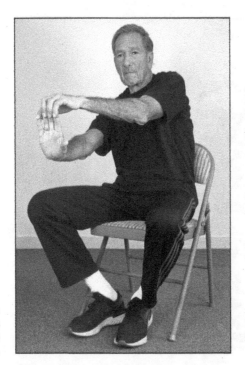

FIGURE 13-14:
Pulling fingers
backward to
stretch the wrist.

IN THE MUDRAS

This chapter has some hand routines that may not seem like Yoga to you, but that couldn't be further from the truth. Yoga has a long-standing tradition of focusing on the hands, hand positions, or gestures. That tradition is referred to as *mudras*.

While mudras may have spiritual roots in certain Eastern religions, in Yoga, mudras are used to affect the mind, a way to direct energy to the brain. In her classic work, *Mudras: Yoga in Your Hands*, author Gertrude Hirschi states: "We can effectively engage and influence our body and our mind by bending, crossing, extending, or touching the fingers with other fingers."

Classic Yoga philosophy sees your hands as having a strong influence on your mind. And, as you attempt to calm your mind by doing poses and movements, performing breath work, or even meditating, your hand position may actually impact your state of mind.

Since hand mudras are typically done while sitting down, Chair Yoga offers you a perfect opportunity to explore this practice.

Chapter **14**

Adding a Chair to Popular Standing and Inversion Poses

U sing a chair in Yoga class isn't a new idea. In fact, chairs have a long history in the studio. The B.K.S. Iyengar tradition of Yoga uses chairs in creative ways to help students get into more traditional poses.

Most of the time, *Chair Yoga* refers to a particular style that allows you to remain seated in a chair while still reaping the benefits of a more traditional Yoga practice. Still, a series of poses does require you to stand or lie near the chair. In these poses, you're using the chair more as a prop, typically to

» Bring the floor closer to you

» Help you maintain balance

» Provide general support — even for nonbalancing poses

REMEMBER

Of course, if you need or want to remain seated while doing Yoga, feel free to skip these poses entirely.

Working on Balance with a Chair by Your Side

Some people are really good at balance, while others struggle. One category of poses is designed to work on your balance, but you do have to come out of your chair in order to use them.

The ultimate goal is not to fall, and having a chair nearby while you attempt a balancing pose can keep you safer. The older you get, the longer it takes to heal from routine injuries. You definitely need to keep your ability to balance in tune — but stay safe while you're doing it. You have to think of your chair as a partner of sorts, whose job it is to help if and when you need it.

REMEMBER

Resist the temptation to think of your chair as a crutch. Rather, it's there like a true partner would be, to support you in times of need. Every Yoga pose offers some kind of physical or emotional benefit. In the case of balancing poses, a chair can help you experience those benefits.

TIP

Good news! Balance can improve with practice. Certainly, building up stabilizing muscles and paying attention to the sensations of balance can help, but practicing is equally important. Stop and think about when you were first learning to ride a bike; it probably felt scary, like it was never going to happen, but it finally did. Your brain learned by paying attention, and your body learned to balance. You just needed to keep at it, and that's what you need now.

Flipping Your Perspective: Inversion Poses

Inversion poses are those where you go upside down or bring your hips higher than your heart. In the Yogic tradition, inversions are believed to offer a host of potential benefits, including the following:

>> Lower heart rate and blood pressure and improved blood flow

>> Reduced stress and tension

>> Improved digestion

>> Greater strength (with improved muscle tone and maybe even some bone)

>> Loosening of tight muscles

>> Supported lymph flow

>> Stimulation of the immune system

>> The opportunity to go inward and explore or calm your mind

>> Improvement in sleep quality

The Yogic body of evidence about inversions is largely anecdotal, but it's certainly persuasive (especially because the practice is thousands of years old). If you're able to get up from your sitting position, we describe a chair inversion at the end of this chapter.

WARNING

Because Yoga inversions require your head to be lower than your hips or heart, they can exacerbate certain health problems, including some retinopathies or glaucoma, high blood pressure, eye issues relating to diabetes, and even some digestive problems like acid reflux or GERD. If these conditions apply to you, check with your doctor; you may need to avoid inversions altogether.

Helping out your heart

The exact ways in which inversions may help the heart is the subject of a lot of clinical studies. What's clear so far is that these poses change the way gravity impacts the body. By putting your legs in the air, with your feet above your heart, gravity helps drain fluid from your legs.

Gaining a lot of relaxation by doing a little

Some inverted poses, such as the reclined inversion in this chapter, are also very restful and may even function as a relaxation period. You may be surprised by how challenging lying there and doing nothing is.

REMEMBER

Never underestimate the importance of just doing nothing — and always resist the urge to skip it. If lying on the ground (or even sitting in your chair) and resting is difficult for you, then that's all the more reason for you to keep practicing it.

Surveying Standing and Inversion Poses Using a Chair for Support

The following poses aren't a complete list of postures you can do with the help of a chair. They are, however, the most popular, and they target all essential areas of your body and mind.

Half forward fold with a chair

Using a chair for support on this pose lets you get your chest parallel to the ground and get a good *hamstring* (the back of your thighs) stretch. It also lengthens the front of your body as well as some of your back muscles.

1. **Stand directly behind your chair and hold on to the back with both hands.**

2. **Take a step back (if necessary) so that your arms are relatively straight.**

3. **On an exhale, fold halfway down so your torso is parallel to the floor (see Figure 14-1).**

    Note: The goal is to do this pose with straight legs, but feel free to bend your knees if necessary.

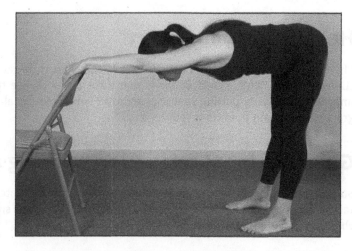

FIGURE 14-1:
Folding forward
with a chair.

4. **Hold this L-shape for about ten breaths.**

5. **On an inhale, rise back up.**

Downward facing dog with a chair

Downward facing dog isn't a resting pose, though it seems like it's used for that in many public classes. This pose not only throws much of your body weight into your shoulders but also may be an inversion if your head sinks below your heart. It's a pose that offers a great way to stretch and strengthen, so deciding whether it's something that should be in your routine is ultimately up to you.

1. **Stand tall directly in front of your chair, facing the seat, with your hands hanging at your sides.**

2. **On an inhale, raise both arms overhead, keeping them straight.**

3. **On your exhale, fold forward from the waist, keeping your back long and flat and bringing the palms of your hands to the seat of the chair (see Figure 14-2).**

   Note: Your ultimate goal is to do this pose with straight legs, but bending your knees a little may make more sense for you.

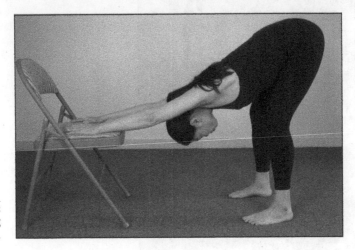

FIGURE 14-2:
Downward facing
dog with a chair.

4. **Hold this pose for six breaths.**

5. **On an inhale, rise back up.**

6. **After you catch your breath (if necessary), repeat Steps 1 through 5.**

Warrior one with a chair

The warrior one pose is a classic Yoga posture that you can do in Chair Yoga either sitting or standing. Although there's currently some debate about how risky having your front knee come over your toes is, keeping your joints *stacked* (your knee directly over your ankle) is practicing on the safe side.

1. **Stand tall behind your chair, placing both hands on the back.**

2. **Step your left foot back and spin it outward about a quarter turn.**

3. On an exhale, bend into your front (right) knee, keeping that knee over your ankle.

4. Lift your right arm up (or both arms, if you want), either straight as shown in Figure 14-3 or bent in a cactus shape.

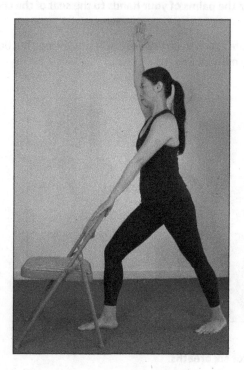

FIGURE 14-3:
Warrior one with
a chair.

5. Hold this pose for six breaths.

6. Lower your arm (or arms) as you slowly straighten your front leg and carefully step out of the pose.

7. Repeat Steps 1 through 6 on the other side.

Warrior two with a chair

Keeping one hand on the chair in this pose is going to provide some added support, but you can also step your back foot back so that it presses against a wall for even more support.

1. Stand tall behind your chair, placing both hands on the back.

2. Step your left foot back and spin it outward about a quarter turn.

3. **On an exhale, bend into the front (right) knee, keeping that knee over your ankle.**

4. **As you inhale, reach your left hand out behind you, straightening your arm and keeping it at shoulder level.**

5. **At the same time, spin your torso to the left (in the same direction your arm is reaching) and open your hips.**

6. **Turn your head toward your right shoulder.**

   See Figure 14-4 for a complete expression of the pose.

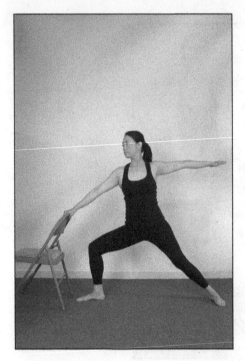

FIGURE 14-4:
Warrior two with
a chair.

7. **Hold this pose for six breaths.**

8. **On an exhale, return to your starting position.**

9. **Repeat Steps 1 through 8 on the other side.**

Standing side kicks with a chair

This routine may remind you of a classic barre exercise professional dancers may do. It's a great way to build some leg strength and stretch some muscles, particularly in the hip. Pay attention to your breath, making this movement a moving meditation, and it becomes definitively Yogic.

1. **Stand tall behind your chair, placing both hands on the back of the chair.**

2. **Shift your weight onto your left leg and raise your right foot slightly off the ground (keeping that right leg straight).**

   Note: Even though you're shifting your weight to one leg, your goal is to remain perfectly upright, keeping your head over your hips and waist.

3. **On an inhale, raise your straight right leg out to the side (see Figure 14-5).**

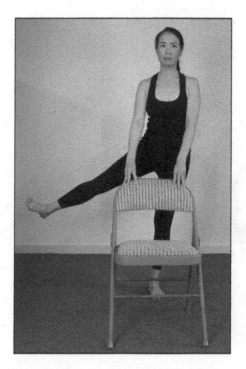

FIGURE 14-5:
Standing side
kicks with a chair.

4. **On your exhale, bring your lifted leg back down.**

5. **Repeat Steps 1 through 4 nine times, moving with your breath.**

6. **Repeat Steps 1 through 5 with the other leg.**

Standing extended side angle with a chair

This posture is an excellent way to stretch out the sides of your body, so take the time to focus on the form. Keep in mind that the chair is there to help you go deeper into the pose so you can reap all the benefits of the posture.

1. **Stand sideways behind your chair with your right side facing the back of the chair.**

2. **Widen your stance a little wider than hip width (2.5 to 3 feet).**

3. **Turn your right toes toward the front and place your right hand on the back of the chair (either the seat or the top).**

4. **On an exhale, bend your right knee and bring your right elbow down to your thigh (still holding on to the chair).**

   Don't let your knee go beyond your ankle in the bend.

5. **Reach your straight left arm overhead along your left ear.**

   See Figure 14-6 for a full expression of the pose.

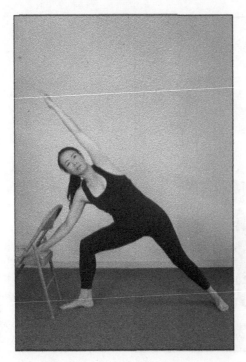

FIGURE 14-6:
Standing
extended side
angle with a
chair.

6. **Hold this pose for six breaths, breathing slowly and smoothly.**

   If possible, breathe through your nose only.

7. **On an inhale, stand back up and lower your arm.**

8. **Spin to the other side of the chair and repeat Steps 1 through 7 on the other side.**

Standing half-moon with a chair

A wall can often be a good way to support your body when attempting this pose. But using a chair has the added advantage of bringing the floor upward so you don't have to reach so far.

1. **Stand with your right side facing the seat of your chair.**

2. **Shift your weight onto your right leg and raise your straight left leg up and out to the side.**

    Aim to get your leg hip height if possible, but if not, do the best you can.

3. **At the same time, reach your straight right arm down, placing the palm of your hand on the seat of the chair (see Figure 14-7).**

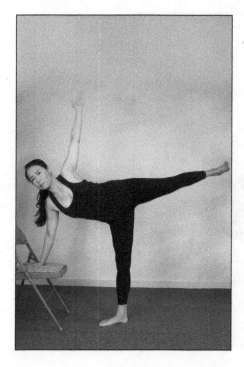

FIGURE 14-7:
Half-moon with a chair.

4. **As you hold the pose, breathe slowly and smoothly for six breaths.**

    Try to breathe through only your nose if possible.

5. **On an exhale, bring your gaze down to your right foot; bring both hands to the seat of your chair and lower your left foot.**

6. On an inhale, stand back up.

7. Repeat Steps 1 through 6 on the other side.

Standing warrior three with a chair

Earlier in this chapter, we cover warrior one and warrior two poses. Warrior three is definitely a balance challenge, so be patient with yourself and be willing to practice in order to strengthen muscles that will ultimately help you in this pose. Using the chair gives you some stabilization as you get deeper into this position that you may not get without the chair.

1. Stand directly behind your chair.

2. Take a step back and inhale.

3. On your exhale, let the palms of your hands rest on the top of your chair, arms extended, as you bend forward into an L-shape.

4. As you inhale, raise your right leg straight behind you, shifting your weight to your left leg and keeping your hips and chest parallel to the ground, and flexing your raised foot (see Figure 14-8).

    Note: Your right hip will want to tilt upward toward the ceiling. Don't let it. Keep your hips square to the ground, even if it means you can't lift your leg as high.

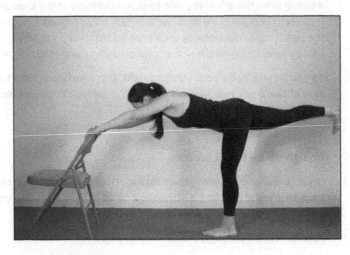

<figure>FIGURE 14-8:
Standing warrior
three with a chair.</figure>

5. Hold this pose for five breaths.

6. On an exhale, lower your leg to the ground, keeping a soft bend in both knees to avoid hyperextension.

7. As you inhale, stand back up.

8. Repeat Steps 1 through 7 on the other side.

Standing tree pose with a chair

This posture may be one of the most popular choices when posing for a picture in front of the Grand Canyon. When you're trying to balance or practicing your balance, using a chair for this pose is just plain smart because having a hand on the chair can help you find your balance. You can then decide to let go if you want to. But it will be nice to know that the chair is always there if you need it.

1. Stand tall on the right side of your chair and hold the back of the chair with your left hand.

2. Shift your weight onto your left leg and then place the sole of your right foot on the inside of your left shin or thigh (above or below the knee joint).

   Because you're placing your foot on the inside of the opposite leg, your knee will be pointing out to the right.

WARNING

   Place your foot above or below the knee joint of the standing leg (on your thigh or your calf). Since the knee is really a hinge joint, it's meant to only go in one direction, forward and back. Not all Yoga teachers, though, agree with this warning since there is some side-to-side movement in the knee and the knee joint often gets pressure from the side. Still, a lot of football players are sitting the bench right now because their knee wasn't meant to go sideways. We recommend erring on the side of caution and staying off the joint.

3. As you inhale, raise your straight right arm overhead (for a full expression of the tree), reaching up toward the ceiling. You can also keep your right hand on your chest or right hip.

   See Figure 14-9.

4. Hold this pose for six breaths.

5. On an exhalation, lower your arm (or arms) and bring your raised foot back to ground (putting a little more bend in that standing leg if you want) and redistribute your weight back to both feet.

6. Repeat Steps 1 through 5 on the other side.

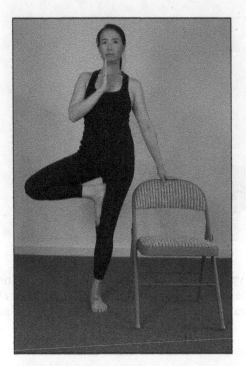

FIGURE 14-9:
Standing tree
pose with a chair.

Inversion: Legs on a chair

Though not a standing pose, this inversion pose does require you to leave your seated position and stretch out on the floor.

Even though inversions offer many potential benefits, as we discuss in the earlier section "Flipping Your Perspective: Inversion Poses," they're often physically challenging. This particular inversion, a variation of a supported shoulder stand, is actually quite easy, though. If you're not careful, you can even fall asleep.

1. **Lie on the ground (or floor) in front of your chair and rest your bent legs on the seat.**

2. **With your straight arms at your sides, turn your hands so your palms are up (see Figure 14-10).**

3. **Relax your body and your mind and just breathe easily.**

   If possible, breathe just through your nose with your mouth gently closed.

4. **Stay motionless in this position for about three to five minutes.**

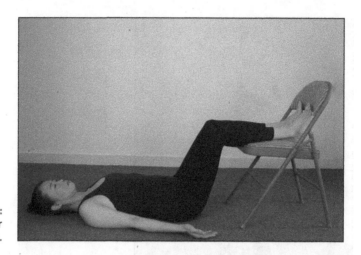

FIGURE 14-10:
Legs on a chair
inversion.

WARNING

When you get back up, roll to one side first, noticing any dizziness. Move slowly as you sit up or come back to your chair. Of course, if you're at all uncomfortable lying down, or if you have a medical condition that lying flat may worsen, skip this pose altogether.

A LONG-STANDING CONCERN

You've heard over and over again about the dangers of immobility, of sitting too much for too long. It's even being called the "new smoking." But how about too much standing? The fact is, if your lifestyle finds you standing for extended periods of time, you could be taxing muscles in your back, legs, feet, and hips.

Of course, standing for long intervals of time is going to occasionally happen, whether you're waiting in line to buy your daily mocha latte or maybe just a few groceries. If, however, your daily routine at home or at work finds you "on your feet all day," you may be inviting pain in the form of sore muscles or even cramps. And this goes for anyone at any age.

To avoid back pain or other types of musculoskeletal problems, your muscles — in this case, particularly, your low-body muscles — should be periodically rested and stretched. If you're setting your phone alarm to make sure you're not sitting at your computer for too long, do the same thing to make sure you're not standing too long, to make sure your muscles are getting some needed rest. Of course, adding Chair Yoga to your daily regime has got to help.

3
Creating Home Routines

Understand the most important principles of Chair Yoga.

Discover routines you can do at your convenience when you only have 15 or 30 minutes to spare.

Pick up some pointers on doing Chair Yoga at your desk.

Try out Chair Yoga even in the tightest spaces.

Pump up your Chair Yoga practice by using hand weights.

Chapter 15

Moving Ahead with Chair Yoga

We offer plenty of sample routines throughout this book to get you started in a Chair Yoga practice. You may even want to dig deeper into the subject or explore Chair Yoga classes at outside venues. As many fitness experts will tell you, regularity is the key to achieving results. That fact is certainly true in Chair Yoga, but you don't have to make it your whole life — just a relatively small part.

REMEMBER

Chair Yoga should ultimately make you feel better, plain and simple. If you have some fun in the process, all the better.

With that in mind, this chapter highlights some of the key points of this style of Yoga that you should keep in mind as you move to a more comprehensive Chair Yoga program.

Perusing Principles of Practice

This chapter highlights some of the critical concepts associated with your Chair Yoga practice. Many of these approaches have already been integrated into the earlier routines, so you may be familiar with some. As you move forward, now, you should take these the principles with you.

REMEMBER

Keep in mind that the ideas listed in this section are not intended to be an onerous set of rules but rather ways to modify your practice to ultimately make it safe, more beneficial, and hopefully more enjoyable.

Just breathing

Yoga in general focuses on the breath, but Chair Yoga may even offer you an opportunity to give your breathing process more attention. By sitting in your chair throughout your practice rather than jumping up and down off of the floor or around your mat, you may find maintaining that breath focus easier.

REMEMBER

Often, easy breathing can be your most powerful tool in controlling stress, anxiety, and even pain. That's why we devote a whole chapter (Chapter 3) to breathing exercises.

TIP

All the sample routines we provide in this book contain breath cues that not only help you coordinate your movement with your breath but also help you breathe in a way that makes it easier to stay relaxed.

Additionally, breath cues help you go more deeply into a pose. So whether you're moving or holding (as we explain in the later section "Embracing the dynamic/static approach"), you're always breathing.

It's not how it looks: Focusing on function over form

Too many Yoga students and teachers let the appearance (*form*) of a pose be more important than its *function*, or overall goal. The bendy (probably hypermobile) Yogi in some book, studio, or video always seems to demonstrate a perfect version of a classic Yoga pose, and then that somehow becomes the benchmark for success. It's all about aesthetics.

But not in Chair Yoga. Chair Yoga is more concerned with what a pose is supposed to do for you — for your body or mind.

Does it give you a stretch that actually feels good or one that goes too far by overstretching a muscle? Is the pose or movement gradually and safely building your muscles or pushing you too quickly, maybe toward injury?

REMEMBER

Pay attention to the signals your body and your mind send you. What Chair Yoga does to nurture you should mean everything.

Embracing the dynamic/static approach

The *dynamic/static approach* — the idea of moving into a pose before holding it — often moves muscles in and out of a pose before going into a static stretch and better protects you from injuries.

Overstretching a muscle can cause hard-to-heal tendon injuries. Such injuries can sideline you for a long time, torpedoing the consistency we discuss earlier in the chapter.

Choosing forgiving limbs

Forgiving limbs (the idea that bending your arms or legs in any pose is okay) is an essential concept in Chair Yoga. Depending on your flexibility, you always have that option (see Figure 15-1b). Make that choice whenever it seems right for your body.

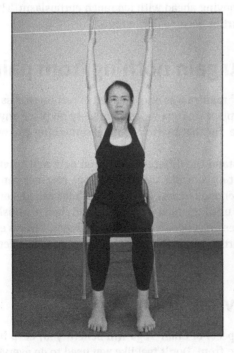 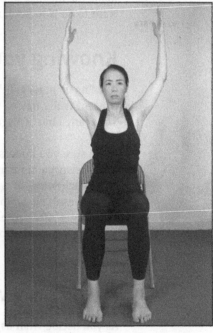

FIGURE 15-1:
Contrasting traditional form (a) with forgiving limbs (b).

REMEMBER

As we note earlier in the chapter, what a pose looks like doesn't matter as long as it's doing something good for you. Opting to bend your arms because a pose is straining your shoulders, or your knees because super-straight legs are hurting your hamstrings, is a sign that you're paying attention to how you feel and to what you need (or don't need) to be comfortable and under control. And you never need to overstretch or strain. You can read more about this concept in the earlier section "It's not how it looks: Focusing on function over form."

Keeping It Real: Starting Chair Yoga with the Right Mindset

Perhaps you're starting Chair Yoga from a place of inactivity, or maybe you already have a Yoga practice but suddenly find that your body doesn't want to do everything it did before. Whatever your reasons for beginning a Chair Yoga regimen, patience is going to be a virtue, both as you try to move into postures and as you look for results.

REMEMBER

As you work to make Chair Yoga a part of your fitness routine and your life, don't make the mistake of moving ahead with *too* much enthusiasm. The last thing you want to do is to get hurt or become discouraged.

Knowing you gain nothing from pain

The "no pain, no gain" mantra was once revered in certain fitness circles, but that concept really has no place in Yoga — and probably no place anywhere. In Chair Yoga (any kind of Yoga, for that matter), pain is something you want to avoid.

TIP

Make sure you understand the difference between pain and soreness. If physical activity isn't a big part of your life, even Chair Yoga routines can make you sore. Muscle soreness, or *working soreness*, as it's sometimes called, comes and goes. It often doesn't show up until the next day or two, and then it vanishes. *Pain*, on the other hand, often comes on suddenly and tends to linger. Always err on the side of avoiding any discomfort if you're not sure whether what you're feeling is soreness or pain.

Doing only what you need

As you decide what aspects of Chair Yoga will benefit you, keep in mind that you have many to choose to from. Don't feel like you need to do everything you see in this book or on some online video. Decide what's best for you.

Anything you decide to skip now is certainly something you can add in later. Some things may never be good for you. That's okay, too. It's your practice and no one else's.

PRIME OF LIFE YOGA

Prime of Life Yoga has its roots in India, where co-author Dr. Larry Payne, under the tutelage of some of Yoga's greatest masters, explored how a Yoga practice can be more accessible to people who are leaving behind their more flexible or more athletic stages of life. This study led Dr. Payne to eventually create Prime of Life Yoga (POLY).

He recalls, "The late professor Sri T. Krishnamacharya is often regarded as the father of modern Yoga. His students included B.K.S. Iyengar; K. Pattabi Jois; Indra Devi; Srivatsa Ramaswami; A.G. Mohan; and his son, my teacher, T.K.V. Desikachar (also now deceased). It was in the early '70s that Krishnamacharya received his first middle-aged Western male student, Dr. Albert Franklin. As Krishnamacharya began working with Dr. Franklin, he started to modify his teachings to make them more accessible to the nontraditional student. This approach was originally called Viniyoga, and I was a charter member of Viniyoga America."

Perhaps no words of Dr. Payne ring more clearly than "You don't have to do the hardest poses to get the benefits of Yoga." That bit of wisdom, along with other POLY tenets, certainly applies to Chair Yoga and should inform how you approach the practice.

Chapter **16**

Fifteen-Minute Routines for Home

I f you're dealing with an all-too-typical schedule, you may have limited time during the course of a day or even a week to devote to your fitness — mental or physical. Don't let those limitations get in your way. Adding 15-minute Chair Yoga routines to your calendar does make a difference.

The following routines are just samples, geared toward beginners and those looking for more advanced movements. Use them as templates to create your own routines. If your needs happen to be very general, you can mix it up from one session to the next.

REMEMBER

Of course, the actual amount of time completing a routine takes you may vary, especially as you become more familiar with the poses, but the benefits are the same.

Beginner Routine

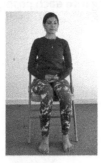

Attunement

1. Sit upright in your chair, letting your head float up toward the ceiling. Even while sitting, try to maintain good posture: your ears over your shoulders and your shoulders over your hips. If you feel stable, close your eyes; if you prefer to keep them open, fix your gaze somewhere on the floor. Allow your breathing to slow as you inhale and exhale through your nose, with your mouth gently shut if possible. (If you need to breathe through your mouth, please do.) Try to let your mind rest, perhaps staying in the present by focusing on your breath. Stay here for about two minutes.

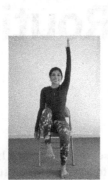

Cross/crawl patterning

2. Still sitting tall, let your arms hang straight at your side. On an inhale, lift your right knee upward, toward your chest, and raise your left hand above your head with a straight arm. Exhale as you lower both your knee and your hand back to the starting position. Repeat this motion on the other side, and then repeat the entire sequence (both sides) five more times, moving with your breath.

   For more information about this pose, see Chapter 1.

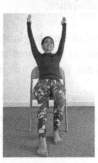

Bent leg arm raise

3. Sit in your chair with your left leg bent and your right leg straight, heel on the ground. Start with your arms at your side, palms down. As you inhale, bring both arms overhead. As you exhale, bring your arms back to your sides. Repeat two more times.

   On an inhale, bring both arms overhead again, but this time keep them overhead as you exhale and then inhale, trying to stretch your arms even further. On your next exhale, bring your arms back down. Repeat this movement for four times and then repeat the sequence on the other side.

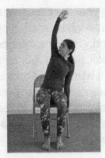

Side bend

4. Sit tall in your chair with your left hand behind your back. On an inhale, reach your right hand toward the ceiling. On your exhale, bend sideways toward the left, bringing that right hand over the top of your head. Try not to let your body tip; stay evenly seated on your chair. As you inhale, sit up straight, reaching your hand up toward the ceiling. Repeat the bending and straightening five times, moving with your breath, and then repeat the sequence on the other side.

Note: The hand that reaches behind you can stay at your low back, or you can hold onto the back of your chair. Also, if you feel unstable, reach down and hold the side of your chair for support instead of bringing that hand behind you.

To find out more about this pose, see Chapter 7.

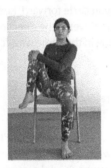

Knee circles

5. Sit tall in your chair with both feet on the ground and take a big inhale. On your exhale, lift your right knee up toward your chest and hold on with both hands. Hold this stretch for about three breaths and drop your left hand, holding onto your knee with just the right. Using your right hand to both support and guide you, circle that knee in one direction for two full breaths. Reverse the direction for two breaths. Lower your right foot back to the ground and repeat the sequence on the other side.

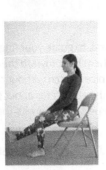

Ankle stretches

6. Sit tall in your chair, rechecking your posture: ears over your shoulders, shoulders over your hips, and both feet flat on the ground. Straighten your right leg, bringing your foot off the ground. As you inhale, point your right foot away from you; as you exhale, pull your foot back toward you. Repeat this movement for a total of three breaths. As you continue to breathe, circle that foot in one direction for a couple of breaths and then reverse the direction for a couple more breaths. Lower your foot back to the ground and repeat the sequence on the other side.

We discuss ankle and feet routines in Chapter 12.

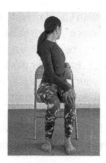

Seated twist (legs forward)

7. Sit upright, making your spine long, with your hands on your thighs. On an inhale, reach for your left knee with your right hand. On your exhale, continue to turn in the same direction, twisting your torso around as your reach your left hand for the back of the chair. Hold this twist (being careful not to overtwist your neck) as you take two to four more breaths. On an exhale, release the twist, turning back around to face the front. Repeat on the other side.

To read more about this pose, flip to Chapter 8.

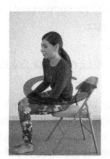

Hip circles

8. Sit toward the front edge of your seat with your feet are flat on the ground or a prop. Be sure to leave space between your back and the back of the chair. Lean forward (hinging from the hips) and start circling your upper torso, breathing in as you circle back and breathing out as you circle forward. Keep circling for a total of six breaths. Reverse the direction of your circle, still breathing in the same way, for a total of six breaths.

To see this pose, refer to Chapter 9.

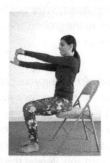

Wrist stretching

9. Sit tall in your chair, keeping your back long and your head reaching toward the ceiling. Extend your right arm in front of you with the palm of your hand facing upward.

Using your left hand, to guide your fingers downward and then to pull them back toward the body, giving your right wrist a nice stretch without causing pain or discomfort. Hold the stretch for about ten breaths and repeat the same sequence with the other wrist.

For more on this stretch, head to Chapter 13.

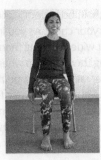

Rest

10. Sit comfortably in your chair (you can sit against the back or cross your legs if you want). If it feels okay, close your eyes; if you prefer to keep them open, just fix your gaze somewhere on the floor. At first, try to keep your mind in the moment. Notice how you're breathing and how much your body likes the air you bring in on your inhales. Maybe use your mind to scan your body to see what feels a little sore or what feels good. Think about your breath. Then allow your mind to either stay focused or wander. Enjoy five minutes of doing nothing.

Advanced Routine

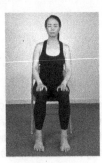

Attunement

1. Sit upright in your chair, letting your head float upward as if being pulled by a magnet. If you feel secure, allow your eyes to close; otherwise, just keep them fixed somewhere on the floor in front of you. Try to slow your breathing, inhaling and exhaling through only your nose, if possible. Let your mind rest, perhaps focusing on your breath. Stay in this relaxed state for two minutes.

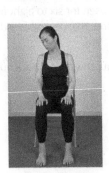

Chin Swings

2. Sit upright, keeping your good posture. Your hands can rest on your legs. Tilt your head down, bringing your chin close to your chest. As you inhale, keep your head tilted down but swing your chin up toward your right shoulder. On your exhale, let your chin drop back down to the center of your chest. On your next inhale, swing your chin up toward your left shoulder, still keeping your head tilted down. On your exhale, let your chin drop back down to the center of your chest. Repeat the sequence six times.

You can read more about this neck routine in Chapter 5.

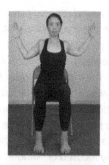

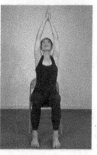

Wing and Prayer

3. Sitting tall in your chair, bring your hands into prayer position in front of your chest. As you inhale, take your bent arms out wide (opening them like wings). As you exhale, bring them back to where you started. On your next inhale, raise your joined hands over your head, keeping your eyes on your fingertips. As you exhale, bring your arms back down. Repeat this sequence five more times, moving with your breath.

Head to Chapter 6 for info on this pose.

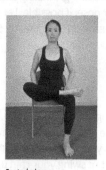

Seated pigeon

4. Sit upright in your chair with your feet on the ground or a prop. Bring your right ankle onto your left knee, crossing your leg. If you feel like you need to intensify the stretch, sit tall as you inhale and lean forward on your exhale (hinging from the hips). Hold whichever position you've chosen for six to eight full breaths and then repeat the stretch on the other side.

To read more about this pose, check out Chapter 9.

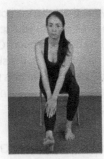

One leg forward bend

5. Sit tall in your chair with your hands on your thighs. As you inhale, extend your right leg straight out with your heel on the floor. Your left foot can come back beneath your chair. Place both your hands on your right thigh. On an exhale, slide both of your hands down your right leg toward your foot as you carefully bend forward. Hold this position for a total of six breaths, and then repeat the sequence on the other side.

To dig into this pose, see Chapter 10.

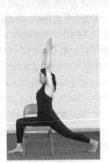

Warrior one with chair

6. Stand tall behind your chair, placing both hands on the back. Step your left foot back and spin it outward about a quarter turn. On an exhale, bend into your front (right) knee, keeping it over your ankle. Lift your right arm up (if you want to), either straight or cactus-shaped. Hold this pose for six breaths and then lower your arm and step out of it. Repeat the sequence on the other side.

This pose is covered in more detail in Chapter 14.

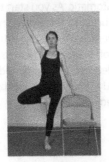

Standing tree pose with a chair

7. Stand tall on the right side of your chair. Hold the back of the chair with your left hand. Shift your weight onto your left leg. Position the sole of your right foot on the inside of your left shin or thigh (above or below the knee joint). Your right knee should be pointing out to the right. As you inhale, Raise your right arm overhead and out to the right (diagonally). Hold this pose for six breaths and then repeat the sequence on the other side.

Chapter 14 has more on this balancing pose.

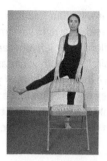

Standing side kicks with a chair.

8. Stand tall behind your chair, placing both hands on the back. Shift your weight onto your left leg and raise your right foot slightly off the ground. On an inhale, raise your straight right leg out to the side. On your exhale, bring it back down. Repeat this movement nine times, moving with your breath and then repeat the entire sequence on the other side.

To take a closer look at this pose, see Chapter 14.

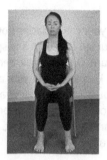

Meditation on the chair.

9. Sit comfortably in your chair (you can sit against the back or cross your legs). If it feels okay, close your eyes; if you prefer to keep them open, fix your gaze somewhere on the floor in front of you. Place your hands on your stomach and feel them rise and fall as you breathe. If it doesn't happen naturally, try to breathe into your stomach, leaving your chest out of the process. You can initially keep your mind from wandering by focusing your attention on the belly breathing you're attempting.

After about 10 to 12 breaths, allow your breathing to become more automatic. As you start to breathe the way you want to breathe, release your mind from any type of confinement, letting it stay with you in the moment or drift off on its own. Remember, if you happen to fall asleep during this period of constructive rest, your body simply needs it, so don't resist or become frustrated.

Chapter **17**

Focusing on a 30-Minute Routine

T hirty minutes is enough time for you to address almost every part of your body (and mind). Think about it: In the time you spend watching a rerun of your favorite sitcom, you can build your muscles, increase your flexibility, and maybe even find an opportunity to relax. All you need is some consistency and some determination to make Chair Yoga part of your routine.

In this chapter, you have a choice between a beginner's and an advanced practitioner's routine. What they have in common is that they're designed to work your entire body. With that said, feel free to pick and choose from the postures and movements that better serve your personal needs. If something causes you discomfort or pain, skip it. If it seems intuitively wrong for you, don't do it. The good news is that any choices you make in this regard don't go on your permanent record.

REMEMBER

Of course, check with your doctor to see whether beginning a fitness regimen is okay for you and whether you should avoid anything in Chair Yoga specifically.

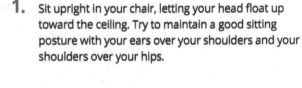

Beginner Routine

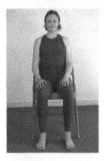

Attunement

1. Sit upright in your chair, letting your head float up toward the ceiling. Try to maintain a good sitting posture with your ears over your shoulders and your shoulders over your hips.

You may close your eyes or fix your gaze somewhere on the floor. Try to slow your breathing, inhaling and exhaling through only your nose if possible.

Sit like this for around two restful minutes.

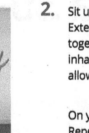

Finger stretch

2. Sit upright in your chair with your feet on the ground. Extend both arms in front of you, with your fingers together and pointed up toward the ceiling. As you inhale, spread your fingers as wide as you can, allowing them to curve a little if they want.

On your exhale, squeeze your fingers into a tight fist. Repeat this opening and closing of your hands five times, moving with your breath.

Chapter 13 has more info on this movement.

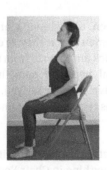

3. Sit upright in your chair with your hands resting comfortably on your thighs. Inhale as you slide your hands up toward your hips, bringing your elbows back (keeping them close to your rib cage).

Allow your back to arch as you tilt your head slightly backward and gaze upward. As you exhale, slide your hands back toward your knees and round your back (like a Halloween cat), allowing your head to tilt slightly forward while looking down.

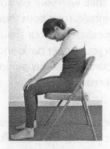

Seated cat/cow

Repeat this back-and-forth movement eight to ten times.

To read more about this movement, see Chapter 7.

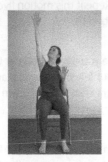

Apple picking

4. Sit tall in your chair, allowing the top of your head to float toward the ceiling. Before you begin reaching upward, your hands can rest palms-down on your thighs or hang at your sides.

As you inhale, reach up with your right hand, pretending to pick an apple from a high branch. On your exhale, bring your right hand back down (to about shoulder level) as you reach up with your left hand.

Repeat this sequence eight times, remembering to move with your breath.

We cover this simple-but-effective movement in Chapter 19.

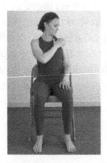

Violin stretch

5. Sit upright in your chair with your ears over your shoulders and the top of your head floating toward the ceiling like it's magnetized. Put your right hand on your left shoulder and look down at your right fingertips.

On an inhale, reach your right hand out to the right, diagonally toward the ceiling. Let your head turn up so your eyes can follow your fingertips.

As you exhale, bring your right hand back down to your left shoulder, keeping your eyes on your right fingertips. Repeat this stretch five times, moving with your breath, and then repeat the entire sequence on the other side.

You can find more info on this movement in Chapter 18.

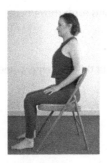

Shoulder shrugs

6. Sit upright in your chair with your ears over your shoulders. As you inhale, raise both shoulders toward your ears. On your exhale, let your shoulders roll back and then fall down your upper back, and return to your starting position. Repeat this motion five times, moving with your breath.

As you inhale, raise both shoulders toward your ears. On your exhale, let your shoulders fall forward, rounding toward your chest and then return to your starting position. Repeat this motion five times, moving with your breath.

As you inhale, raise your right shoulder toward your right ear. Leave your left shoulder in place. On your exhale, let your right shoulder fall down your back and return to your starting position.

Repeat this motion with your left shoulder, and then repeat the right-then-left sequence five times.

Chapter 6 has more on this stretch.

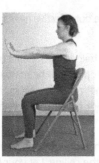

Flexing and extending your wrists

7. Sit upright in your chair with your feet on the ground. Extend both arms in front of you parallel to the ground, holding your fingers together. As you inhale, point your fingers upward bringing your wrist into extension. On your exhale, swing your fingers downward so they point toward the ground, bringing your wrists into flexion. Repeat this up-and-down motion five times, moving with your breath.

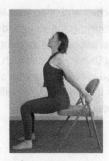

Seated camel pose

8. Sit upright in your chair, lengthening your spine by allowing the top of your head to rise toward the ceiling. As you inhale, reach behind you with both hands and grab the chair, slightly tilting your head backward and looking up toward the ceiling. *Note:* Don't tilt your head back too far.

Hold this pose for six to eight breaths.

You find out more about this pose in Chapter 7.

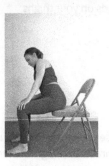

Hip circles

9. Sit in your chair toward the front edge of your seat; this should help ensure that your feet are flat on the ground (or a prop, if you're using one). Be sure to leave space between your back and the back of the chair.

Lean forward a bit (hinging from the hips) and circle your upper torso in a continuous movement, breathing in as you circle back and breathing out as you circle forward. Keep circling with this breathing pattern for five more breaths.

Reverse the direction of your circle, still breathing the same way. Keep circling with this breathing pattern for five more breaths. Close your eyes during this routine if you feel stable.

Read more about this movement by going to Chapter 7.

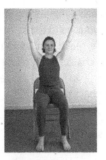

10. Sit upright in your chair and open your legs to about hip width. Let your arms hang straight down at your sides. As you inhale, sweep your straight arms out to the sides and bring them overhead with palms facing one another. As you exhale, bring your straight arms down outside your legs and fold over, allowing your head to drop between your legs.

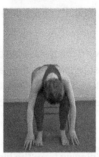

Note: If you have any issues that would be worsened by dropping your head, only bend down halfway, keeping your hands on your thighs.

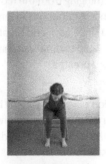

As you inhale, raise your torso halfway up so your back is flat and parallel to the ground and spread your arms straight out to the side like you're an airplane; bring your head up, gazing forward. On an exhale, drop your head and arms back into the forward fold.

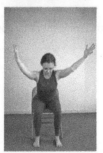

On your inhale, reach up as you come into a squat; you can stay seated, pressing your feet into the ground, or lift your seat just off of your chair. On an exhale, come back to the starting position, sitting tall in your seat with your arms dropped to the sides. Repeat the entire sequence four to six times.

Chapter 1 has more details on this flow.

Seated rejuvenation sequence

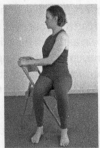

Seated twist

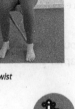

REMEMBER

11. Sit in your chair with your hands resting on your thighs. As you inhale, let your head float toward the ceiling giving you a long back.

On your exhale, twist your entire torso to the right, bringing your right hand to the back of the chair to help deepen the twist (if you can't reach the back of the chair, reach anywhere behind you). Hold the pose for five more breaths, continuing to breathe.

This is a torso twist; resist the urge to twist with your neck.

Release the twist on an exhale, bringing your body back around to the starting position. Repeat on the other side.

To discover more about this pose, head to Chapter 8.

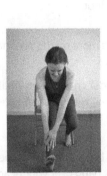

One-leg hamstring stretch

12. Sit upright in your chair with your hands on your thighs. As you inhale, extend your right leg straight out with your heel on the floor. On an exhale, slide both of your hands down your right leg toward your foot as you carefully bend forward.

Note: Your tight hamstring is probably what prevents you from bending as far forward as you want to go. Don't try to compensate by forcing your back to bend farther. And don't round forward if it causes you pain or discomfort.

Hold this position for a total of six breaths. Repeat on the other side.

Chapter 10 has details on this pose.

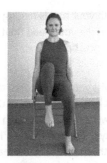
Seated march

13. Sit upright in your chair with your hands resting on your thighs. March in your seat, bringing one knee up and down and then the other. Continue this marching movement, breathing as normally as possible (when your breathing starts to become labored, that's your signal to stop).

You can find out more about this routine by looking to Chapter 9.

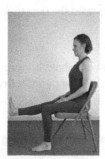
Ankle circles

14. Sit upright with a long back and your feet on the ground. Extend your right leg straight out in front of you. Circle your ankle to the right for five breaths, breathing gently (and through your nose only, if possible).

Change the circling direction to the left and repeat the movement. Then repeat the sequence with the other foot.

Chapter 12 has more on this routine.

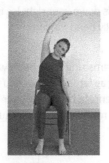
Seated side bends

15. Sit upright in your chair. On an inhale, grab the side of your chair with your left hand and raise your right arm toward the ceiling.

As you exhale, bend sideways to the left and bring that right hand over your head in the same direction. ***Note:*** With your body leaning left, you may feel yourself tipping sideways. Try to bring yourself back down into the chair so that you're sitting with an even amount of pressure on both sides.

Hold the side bend for about six breaths total. Repeat on the other side.

Read more about side bends in Chapter 7.

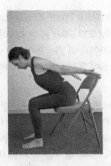

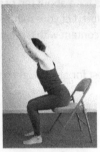

Seated thunderbolt

16. Sit tall in your chair with your arms hanging straight at your sides. On an exhale, lean forward (without rounding your back) and bring your straight arms up behind you. As you inhale, swing your arms forward and up. You can stay seated and push your feet into the floor or actually lift your buttocks off of the chair. (Either engages the same leg muscles you'd use to squat.)

As you exhale, lower your arms, come back to your seat (if you lifted), and return to the bent-forward position. Repeat this up-and-down sequence five times, moving with your breath.

You can discover more about this routine in Chapter 18.

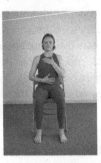

Deep breathing routine

17. Sit upright in your chair with your head over your shoulders. Place your right hand on your stomach and your left hand on your chest. Inhale deeply through your nose and notice where you feel like the air is flowing — more into your stomach? Your chest? Both? Exhale deeply through your nose. Continue this pattern of breathing for about ten more breaths.

Chapter 3 has information on this routine that's intended to keep your mind focused on your breath.

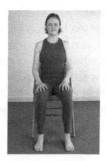

Meditation and rest

18. Get comfortable in your chair. Close your eyes if doing so feels okay and slow your breathing — in and out through your nose. (If you feel too unstable with your eyes closed, just stare down at the floor.)

As you inhale, visualize that you feel lighter. As you exhale, visualize that you're starting to float upward. Continue this visualization, imagining yourself to be lighter and lighter, floating higher and higher. Maintain this focus for a about ten breaths and then don't make any effort. Let your mind remain stable or journey off, being content with either.

Continue to just rest for about eight to ten minutes.

Advanced Routine

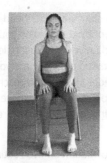

Attunement

1. Sit upright in your chair, letting your head float up toward the ceiling. Try to maintain a good sitting posture with your ears over your shoulders and your shoulders over hips. You may close your eyes or fix your gaze somewhere on the floor. Try to slow your breathing, inhaling and exhaling through only your nose if possible.

Maintain this position for two or three minutes.

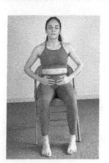

Belly breathing

2. Sit upright in your chair with your head over your shoulders. Place both hands comfortably on your stomach. Inhale through your nose, feeling your stomach rise. Exhale through your nose, feeling your stomach deflate. Repeat this sequence for a total of eight breaths.

We cover this breathing technique in Chapter 3.

3. Sit upright as tall as you can. Your hands can rest on your legs and your feet should rest comfortably on the floor or a prop.

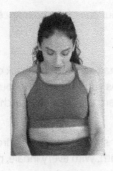

On an exhale, tilt your head down, bringing your chin gently to your chest. As you inhale, bring your chin back up to the starting position. Repeat this sequence twice, moving with your breath, and then again, holding your chin down for six seconds. As you inhale, bring your chin back up.

Sit tall with your chin level. Take a big inhale. As you exhale, rotate your head to the right, keeping your chin level. On your inhale, rotate your chin back to the starting position. Repeat this movement twice, moving with your breath, and then again, holding your rotation for six seconds.

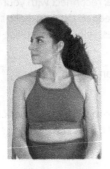

On your next inhale, rotate your chin to the starting position. Repeat the sequence in the opposite direction.

Sitting comfortably but maintaining a good posture, take in a big inhale. As you exhale, tilt your head to the right, keeping your chin up.

Note: You may be inclined to lean your whole body in the direction of the tilt. Try not to.

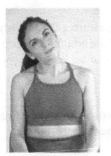

Neck sequence

As you inhale, tilt your head back to the starting position. Repeat this sequence twice, moving with your breath, and then again, holding your tilt for six seconds. On your next inhale, tilt your head back up to the starting position. Repeat the sequence in the opposite direction.

For a more complete discussion of these routines, see Chapter 5.

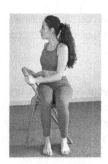

Seated twist (sideways)

4. Sit sideways in your chair with your knees out to the right.

As you inhale, sit tall and grab the back of your chair (don't twist yet). As you exhale, twist your torso so you're facing toward the back of your chair.

Hold this twist for six full breaths. Ensure you aren't holding your breath. With every inhale, make sure your head is floating upward and your spine is long. With every exhale, reconnect with your twist — maybe twisting deeper. On an exhale, spin back toward your knees, releasing the twist.

Repeat the twist on the other side.

WARNING

This isn't a routine to stretch your neck. Looking back in the direction of the twist may make sense, but don't overtwist.

Head to Chapter 18 for more on this routine.

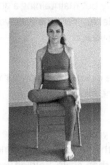

Seated pigeon

5. Turn your chair back around. Sit upright in your chair with your feet on the ground or a prop. Bring your right ankle onto your left knee with your right foot flexed.

Note: If this movement is painful for you or causes discomfort, just don't do this pose.

TIP

Totally optional addition: If you feel like you need a deeper stretch, sit tall as you inhale and lean forward on your exhale. Bending forward from the hips instead of rounding your spine increases the intensity of the stretch. But remember: Don't do it if it hurts.

Hold your cross-legged position for five more breaths. Repeat the sequence on the other side.

You can read about this particular variation of seated pigeon in Chapter 9.

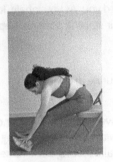

Seated forward fold (both legs straight)

6. Sit tall in your chair; slide to the front edge of your seat so your feet can rest firmly on the ground. Open your feet and knees to about hip width. On an inhale, reach your straight arms up and overhead. As you exhale, bring your arms and head down so that your head is between your knees and your arms are outside your legs, hands reaching toward the floor.

Relax your neck, letting your head fall toward the floor. Hold the fold for six breaths. On an inhale, slowly come back up (using your hands on your knees as leverage if you want).

WARNING

If you have a medical condition that doesn't allow you to let your head to fall below your hips, you can keep your back straight (instead of rounding it) and not let your head fall below your knees. To be on the safe side, you may want to skip this pose entirely.

For more information about this exercise, see Chapter 18.

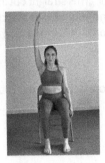

Arm raises

7. Sit tall with both feet on the ground. Raise your right arm in front of you and overhead on an inhale. Lower your arm on the exhale. Repeat with your left arm.

On your next inhale, raise both arms in front of you and overhead. On your exhale, lower both arms. Repeat the entire sequence (right arm, left arm, and both arms) five times.

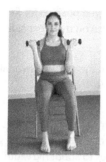

Seated bicep curls with weights

8. Sit tall in your chair with both feet on the ground or a prop. Place your hands comfortably on your thighs while gripping your weights with your palms facing up.

   On an exhale, bend your arms as you bring the weights up toward you. As you inhale, lower your arms back to your starting position. Repeat for a total of 10 to 15 reps.

   Check out this routine in Chapter 20.

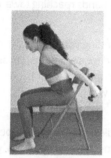

Seated triceps pulses with weights

9. Still gripping the weights, sit tall in your chair and lean slightly forward with your arms hanging straight down and your palms facing back. Raise your straight arms behind you until you feel some natural resistance.

   Making sure you're still breathing, pulse your arms upward, feeling the tension in the back of your upper arms. Continue to pulse, breathing normally, for about five breaths.

   You can read more about this routine in Chapter 20.

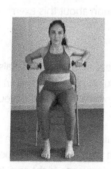

Seated rows with weights

10. Sit tall in your chair, gripping the weights at armpit level with your elbows pointing straight back. On an inhale, extend your arms straight out in front of you. As you exhale, bend your elbows and come back to the starting position. Repeat for a total of eight to ten reps.

    Chapter 20 has more details on this routine.

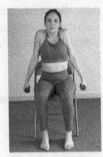

Seated shrugs with weights

11. Sit tall in your chair with your weights in your hands and your arms hanging straight down at your sides, palms facing inward. On an inhale, lift your shoulders up toward your ears, keeping your arms hanging.

As you exhale, lower your shoulders so you're back to your starting position. Repeat for a total of 10 to 15 reps.

You can read up on this routine in Chapter 20.

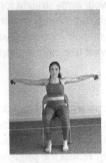

Seated flies

12. Sit tall in your chair with your weights in your hands and your arms hanging straight down at your sides, palms facing inward. On an inhale, bring your straight arms up to shoulder level, making a T-shape. As you exhale, lower your straight arms back to the starting position. Repeat for a total of eight to ten reps.

Find out more about this routine in Chapter 20.

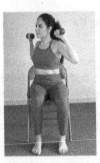

Seated twist with weights

13. Sit tall in your chair, gripping the weights in your hands. Bend your elbows and raise your arms so that your weights are resting just above your shoulders. Take a big inhale; on your exhale, rotate your torso all the way to the left. Inhale as you turn back around (to your starting position).

On your exhale, rotate your torso all the way to the right. Following your breath, keep rotating back and forth until you've done eight to ten rotations on each side.

You can check out this routine in Chapter 20.

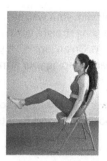

Chair Yoga boat pose

14. Sit upright in your chair, sliding forward a bit to leave space behind you. Grip the sides of your chair seat with both hands. Raise both knees in the air and lean back.

Note: You can lift one leg at a time if that makes more sense.

TIP

Totally optional addition: Let go of the sides of the chair and extend your arms straight forward. However, if you feel this move is compromising your posture, causing you pain, or leading you to hold your breath, you may want to continue gripping the chair for support.

Try to straighten your leg or legs (but don't worry if you can't). Make sure you're still breathing. Hold the pose for two to four breaths. Lower your leg(s). If you chose to do one leg, repeat the sequence with the other leg.

Flip to Chapter 8 for this routine.

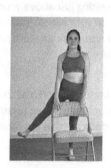

Chair Yoga side kicks

15. Stand tall behind your chair with your head over your hips and feet. Place both hands on the back of the chair. Shift your weight onto your left leg and raise your right foot slightly off the ground (keeping that right leg straight). On an inhale, raise your straight right leg out to the side.

On your exhale, bring it back down. Repeat this movement nine times, moving with your breath. Switch to the other side and repeat the sequence.

Chapter 14 has more on this routine.

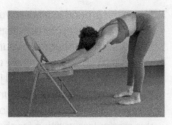
Downward facing dog with a chair

16. Stand tall directly in front of your chair, facing the seat, with your hands hanging at your sides. On an inhale, raise both arms overhead, keeping your arms straight. On your exhale, fold forward from the waist, keeping your back long and flat and bringing the palms of your hands to the seat of the chair.

Note: Your ultimate goal is to do this pose with straight legs, but putting a little bend in your knees may make more sense.

Hold this pose for six breaths. As you inhale, rise back up (bending your knees any amount you want).

Head to Chapter 14 for this pose.

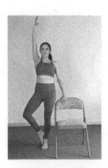
Chair Yoga tree pose (standing)

17. Stand tall on the right side of your chair. Hold the back of the chair with your left hand. Shift your weight onto your left leg while you place the sole of your right foot on the inside of your left shin or thigh (above or below the knee joint).

Your knee will be pointing out to the right. As you inhale, raise your straight right arm overhead, reaching up toward the ceiling. Hold this pose for six breaths.

On an exhale, with a slight bend in your left knee, lower your arms and bring your right foot back to the ground so you're standing evenly on both feet. Repeat the sequence on the other side.

To read more about this pose, see Chapter 14.

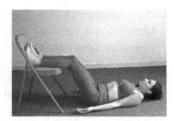

Chair Yoga inversion

18. Lie on the ground in front of your chair and rest the calves of your bent legs on the seat. With your straight arms at your sides, turn your hands so your palms are up. Relax your body and your mind and just breathe easily (if possible, through your nose only and with your mouth gently closed). Stay in this motionless position for about six to eight minutes (longer if you want).

WARNING

When you get back up, roll to one side first, noticing any dizziness. Move slowly as you sit up or come back to your chair. If you're at all uncomfortable lying down, or if you have some kind of medical condition that would be worsened by lying flat with your legs above you, skip this pose all together.

Chapter **18**

Working in Yoga at Your Desk

E ven though sitting too much can be detrimental to overall health, many people find themselves chained to their desks, hunched toward a computer for hours at a time. That's a recipe for disaster — or at least tension — especially for your neck, shoulders, and even your back and hips.

That's where doing Chair Yoga at your desk comes in.

REMEMBER

In Chair Yoga, your chair needs to be your partner and offer you a sense of stability and support. If your desk chair rolls or swivels, it may be more of a hindrance than a helper. Find a sturdy, stationary chair specifically for your Chair Yoga practice and have it nearby to make a quick switch before you begin your routines.

Sneaking in Chair Yoga for a Physical and Mental Break

When you're busy at your desk, sometimes jumping up and running off to the gym or a Yoga class is just unrealistic. Still, your body desperately needs the movement, the opportunity to stretch.

Taking a short break and doing a desk Yoga routine, right in your chair, offers many benefits, including

>> Stretching tight or immobile muscles

>> Reducing stress and tension

>> Increasing the ability to focus on the task at hand, which ultimately increases productivity

>> Improving digestion (which can be compromised by extended sitting)

REMEMBER

Of course, proper ergonomics — your physical setup, your keyboard and monitor height, and so on — are also essential, but that's a topic for another book.

Clocking in for Chair Yoga at Your Desk

You can do almost every pose in this book while sitting at your desk. When you're plopped down at your desk for extended periods of time, your, neck, shoulders, and hands/wrists become particularly susceptible to tightness or tension. Spending a lot of time on your computer, for example, means your wrists may be vulnerable to repetitive motion injury (such as carpal tunnel syndrome). You may want to check out the chapters that focus on these areas of the body in particular:

>> Neck: Chapter 5

>> Shoulders: Chapter 6

>> Hands and wrists: Chapter 13

In addition to the exercises in other chapters, the following sections offer some other good routines you can do while sitting at your desk.

Searching for hot spots

The following routine embraces the value of self-massage in Yoga.

TECHNICAL STUFF

Yoga is sometimes considered a sister science of *ayurveda*, an ancient, holistic approach to healing. Ayurveda has its roots in India and is known for its own use of self-massage — a technique called *abhyanga*.

1. **Sit upright in your chair.**

2. **Use the fingers of your right hand to search the muscles of your left shoulder for tender points, particularly knots (see Figure 18-1).**

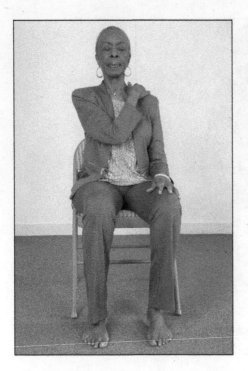

FIGURE 18-1:
Searching for hot
spots.

3. If you find a knot, grab and squeeze the area with your fingers.

4. Release the pressure and begin to gently massage the area with long, soft strokes.

5. Repeat Steps 2 through 4 on the other side.

The violinist stretch

This simple stretch can be a very effective way to loosen tight neck and shoulder muscles.

1. Sit upright in your chair with your ears over your shoulders and the top of your head being drawn toward the ceiling like it's magnetized.

2. Put your right hand on your left shoulder and look down at your right fingertips (see Figure 18-2).

3. On an inhale, raise your right hand diagonally out to the right toward the ceiling, turning your head turn so your eyes can follow your fingertips (see Figure 18-3).

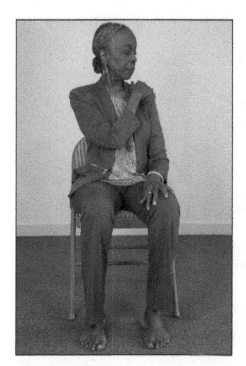

FIGURE 18-2:
Hand on
shoulder.

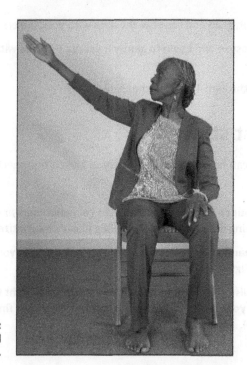

FIGURE 18-3:
Hand
reaches out.

4. As you exhale, bring your right hand back down to your left shoulder (returning to where you started), keeping your eyes on your fingertips.

5. Repeat Steps 3 and 4 five times, moving with your breath.

6. Repeat Steps 2 through 5 on the other side.

Seated twist for work

This routine is a slight variation on the seated twist in Chapter 8.

The main target is the torso, although it also adjusts your spine. At some point in your day, you'll twist your body — maybe while spinning around to see who tapped you on the shoulder or reaching for some paperwork on the table behind you. Twisting routines help prepare your body for that sudden movement and maybe even prevent a pull or strain.

1. Sit sideways in your chair, with your ears over your shoulders and your knees off to the right (see Figure 18-4).

2. As you inhale, grab the back of your chair without twisting (see Figure 18-5).

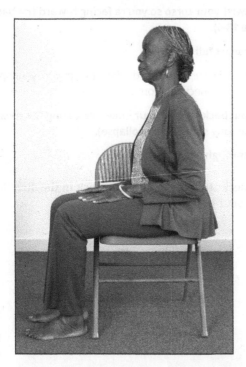

FIGURE 18-4:
Sitting sideways.

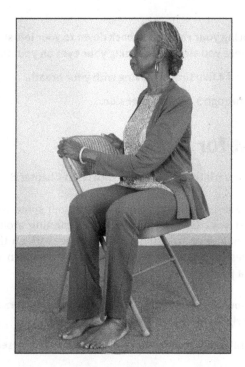

FIGURE 18-5:
Holding the back
of the chair.

3. **As you exhale, twist your torso so you're facing toward the back of your chair (see Figure 18-6).**

4. **Hold this twist for six full breaths.**

   With every inhale, make sure your head is floating upward, your spine long. With every exhale, reconnect with your twist — maybe twisting deeper.

5. **On an exhale, spin back toward your knees, releasing the twist and maintaining your long spine (don't collapse).**

6. **Repeat Steps 1 through 5 on the other side.**

This routine isn't a neck stretch. You can look back in the direction of the twist, but don't over-twist your neck.

WARNING

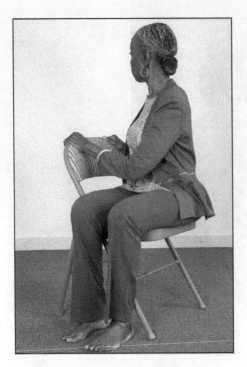

FIGURE 18-6:
Twisting in the
chair.

Chest and shoulder stretch

This stretch is actually great for your hands and wrists, low back, and hips. Your range of motion may be limited at first, but that changes as you continue to practice

WARNING

Because this movement involves dropping your head, it may aggravate certain conditions. If you're at all uncertain, don't drop your head too low. You can even skip this routine entirely.

1. **Sit tall near the front edge of your chair (to make some space behind you) with your feet on the ground and your hands clasped behind you (see Figure 18-7).**

    Note: If you can't clasp your hands, use a dish towel or strap as Figure 18-8 illustrates.

2. **Inhale, and then as you exhale, bend forward and raise your arms up behind you (see Figure 18-9).**

    You want your arms to be as straight as possible in this stretch, but depending on your chair, you may need to bend them initially so that your hands clear the back of the chair.

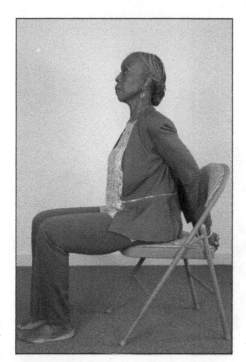

FIGURE 18-7:
Clasping your
hands.

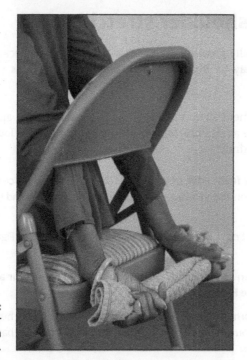

FIGURE 18-8:
Joining your
hands with a
towel.

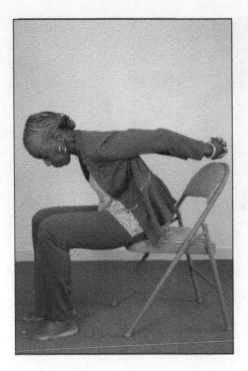

FIGURE 18-9:
Folding forward.

3. On an inhale, rise back up to your starting position.

4. If you feel like another stretch, repeat Steps 2 and 3.

Chair thunderbolt variation

This pose is a chair adaptation of a classic Yoga move. It's a great way to loosen up your whole body and maybe even build some strength along the way.

1. Sit tall in your chair with your arms hanging straight at your sides (see Figure 18-10).

2. On an exhale, lean forward (without rounding your back) and bring your straight arms up behind you (see Figure 18-11).

3. As you inhale, swing your straight arms forward and up over your head, pushing your feet into the floor (see Figure 18-12).

   Note: If you prefer, you can lift your buttocks off the chair and come into a squat. Either version engages the same leg muscles.

4. As you exhale, lower your arms, come back to your seat if you lifted off, and return to the bent-forward position in Step 2.

5. Repeat Steps 3 and 4 five times, moving with your breath.

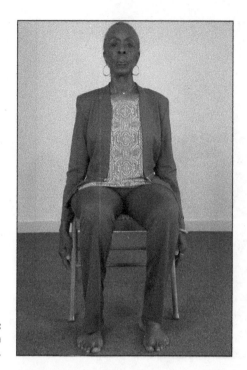

FIGURE 18-10:
Sitting with
straight arms.

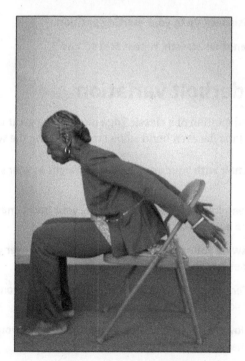

FIGURE 18-11:
Leaning forward
with straight
arms behind you.

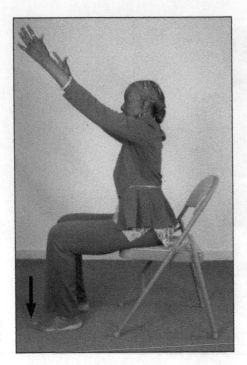

FIGURE 18-12:
Arms swing
upward.

Forward fold in a chair

A simple forward fold offers many benefits, including decompressing the spine. Basically, what you start to accomplish in this position is reversing the pull of gravity. When you're upright, gravity actually pulls the vertebrae in your spine downward. A forward fold allows your vertebrae to separate a bit, perhaps releasing some pressure or tension.

REMEMBER

Your spine not only includes your upper and lower back but also extends into your neck (your *cervical spine*).

WARNING

This pose can exacerbate some conditions, such as unchecked high blood pressure, vertigo, retinopathy, and even a sore back. If you have such a condition, or just an aversion to dropping your head below your hips, you may want to keep your back straight (instead of rounding it) and not let your head fall below your knees. Of course, you may also want to skip this pose entirely.

1. Sit tall in your chair, sliding to the front edge of your seat so your feet can rest firmly on the ground.

2. Open your feet and knees to about hip width (see Figure 18-13).

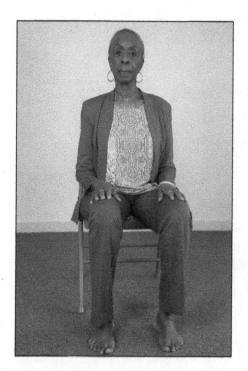

FIGURE 18-13:
Sitting with your
knees open.

3. On an inhale, reach your straight arms up and overhead.

4. As you exhale, bend forward so your head is between your knees and your arms are outside your legs, hands reaching toward the floor (see Figure 18-14).

TIP

If you happen to have a desk directly in front of you blocking your forward bend, just rest your head on your folded arms right on your desk. By relaxing all the muscles in your neck and shoulders while you do this step, it can still be a very effective way to release tension.

5. Relax your neck, letting your head fall toward the floor.

6. Hold the fold for six breaths.

7. On an inhale, slowly come back up (using your hands on your knees as leverage if you want).

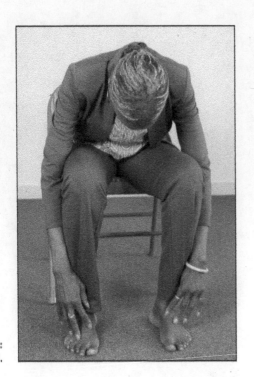

FIGURE 18-14:
Folding forward.

Chapter **19**

Chair Yoga in Transit

n general, Yoga doesn't require a lot of space; you don't practice on a Yoga court or Yoga field. For the most part, you just need a relatively small mat — or a chair.

Sometimes, however, you may find yourself restrained in surroundings that are a bit tight even for Yoga. Fortunately, Chair Yoga offers some powerful routines that don't demand much room — just thoughtfulness and perhaps a little dedication. Some routines in other chapters fit this bill, but this chapter offers new movements for you to consider.

REMEMBER

The space requirements for Chair Yoga may be small, but the potential benefits are huge for both your body and your state of mind.

Benefitting from Yoga Near or Far, on a Plane or in a Car

Whether you're on a bucket-list vacation or just a weekend road trip, traveling can be stressful. It can keep you tense and immobile — two things that work against your goal to be healthy and relaxed. Maybe you're dealing with a cramped middle seat on an airplane, or perhaps you're surrounded on all sides by fellow passengers who don't seem too worried about your comfort level.

Chair Yoga can help. Why bring your Chair Yoga practice with you on a trip?

>> It doesn't take up any room in your suitcase because it's all in your head.

>> It requires you to think about your breathing, and breathing helps you relax.

>> It counteracts the damage from too much sitting by loosening stiff muscles and joints that can lead to discomfort or even pain.

>> It allows you some essential movement while respecting the personal space of people around you.

>> It's a perfect place to meditate — and you probably have the time. (Unless you're the driver or the pilot. . .)

REMEMBER

Meditation, breath work, and thoughtful movement can be an antidote for so much of the mental and physical stress associated with traveling. You don't have to be destined for some holistic wellness resort in order to bring a degree of fitness into your plane, bus, train, or car seat.

Taking on Chair Yoga in Tight Places

Here are some good Chair Yoga routines you can do in compact spaces, including while traveling. These movements target anxiety, as well as tightness in your neck, shoulders, back, hips, legs, and feet.

Apple picking stretch

This movement may require a little imagination, but it's easy to do, and the stretch feels great.

1. **Sit tall in your seat, allowing the top of your head to float toward the ceiling.**

    Your hands can rest palms-down on your thighs or hang at your sides.

2. **As you inhale, reach up with your right hand, pretending to pick an apple off a high branch (see Figure 19-1).**

    While your eyes may naturally look upward as you imagine this activity, it's best to keep your eyes looking forward so you don't hold your head back for an extended period of time.

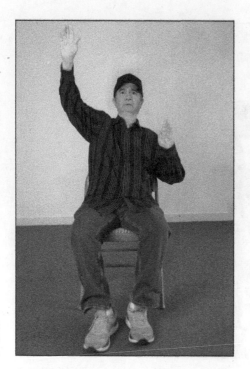

FIGURE 19-1:
Picking an
imaginary apple.

3. On your exhalation, lower your right hand to wherever it feels natural, and raise your left arm overhead, again mimicking the apple picking action.

4. Repeat this sequence, alternating right and left, seven more times (remember to move with your breath).

Seated rowing

This exercise helps you stretch your arms in a small space.

1. Sit tall in your seat with your arms extended straight out and your hands in with your palms down (see Figure 19-2).

2. As you inhale, pull your arms toward you, bending your elbows and sending them backward (see Figure 19-3).

3. On your exhale, extend your arms back out to the starting position.

4. Repeat Steps 2 and 3, moving with your breath, 15 to 20 times.

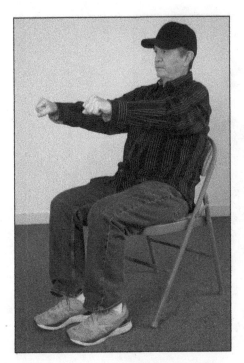

FIGURE 19-2:
Preparing to row.

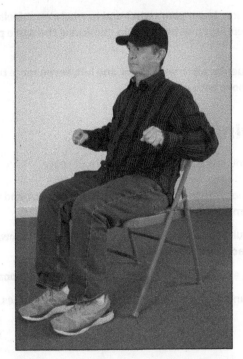

FIGURE 19-3:
Pulling the
imaginary oar.

Knee to elbow

Although this movement provides a nice stretch, it also engages some large muscles and increases circulation.

1. **Sit tall in your chair with your hands behind your neck (see Figure 19-4).**

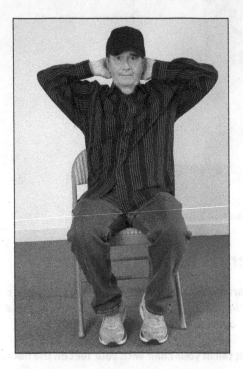

2. **On your exhale, lean forward, bringing your right elbow toward your left knee (see Figure 19-5).**

    Note: If you're able, you can lift your knee toward that elbow, lifting your left foot off the ground.

3. **As you inhale, sit back up into your starting position.**

4. **On your exhale, lean forward, bringing your left elbow toward your right knee.**

    Note: Again, lift your knee toward your elbow, if you're able.

5. **As you inhale, sit back up into your starting position.**

6. **Repeat Steps 2 through 5 five times, moving with your breath.**

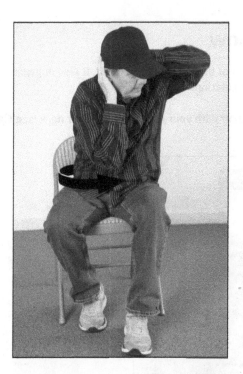

FIGURE 19-5:
Knee to elbow.

Forward bends for tight spaces

This forward bend variation is the perfect movement when you're stuck in a seat. Pay particular attention to the breath cues, which should make this movement easier and ultimately allow for more repetitions.

1. As you inhale, sit tall in your chair with your feet on the floor.

2. On your exhale, bend forward, hinging from the hips, as you raise your heels (see Figure 19-6).

3. On your inhale, lower your heels back to the ground and sit back up (hinging from the hips and returning to your starting position).

4. Repeat Steps 2 and 3 nine times, moving with your breath.

WARNING

Letting your head go when you bend forward can be a great way to release tension in your neck, but make sure other conditions you may have don't prohibit you from doing this movement.

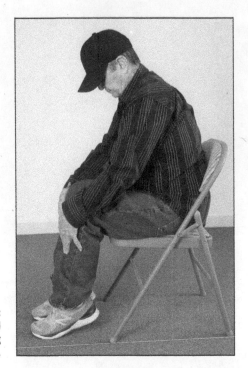

FIGURE 19-6:
Bend forward
while raising
heels.

CHAIR YOGA ON A PLANE

The first time Larry Payne taught Chair Yoga was decades ago, on a private plane flying across the Arctic Ocean:

"I was invited by the World Presidents' Organization (WPO) to be the Yoga teacher on a Russian nuclear icebreaker. The whole excursion was primarily to hold a black-tie dinner on board the ship, at the North Pole.

The list of attendees consisted of many of the wealthiest people in the world, including the late John Templeton, founder of the Templeton Fund. People arrived from all parts of the United States, taking this private jet to Murmansk, Russia, where we would board the icebreaker for the North Pole. It was on this plane trip, which included about 25 couples, that I was asked to lead the passengers in some kind of Yoga routine. I did a class consisting of ten poses, and almost everybody participated, sitting right there in the seats of the plane."

Chapter **20**

Sit Up and Weight: Adding Weights to Your Chair Yoga

Traditional Yoga routines typically don't require using things like dumbbells to add weight-resistance to a pose. In Yoga, you actually build muscle by working against your own body weight.

Adding additional weight to the equation can both intensify and accelerate the muscle-building aspects of Yoga. Of course, you can just supplement your Yoga practice with other types of exercise on other days. However, incorporating weights directly into Chair Yoga creates a sort of hybrid routine. In this chapter, we look at some of the basics for adding weights to your Chair Yoga practice and provide some poses you can try with weights.

Weighing the Fundamentals of Adding Weights to Your Chair Yoga

TIP

If going out to the gym or participating in another kind of physical fitness activity is problematic for you, you may want to consider adding weights to your Chair Yoga routine, even if it's only for a few poses.

Doing Chair Yoga with weights can actually enhance some of its, including the following:

» **Increased muscle mass:** Adding weights to your routine may build muscles faster, and those muscles can help support potentially problematic structures like your back or knees. As well as improving your posture, toned muscles can help with balance and maintaining a healthy weight.

» **Greater bone density:** Resistance training can result in increased bone density, or at least slow down the general bone loss that occurs over time. And even if you think you're still too young to worry about decreased bone density, now is the perfect time to confront the problem, regardless of your age.

The following sections explore some aspects of doing Chair Yoga with weights to help set you off on the right foot.

I don't own dumbbells: Expanding your view of "weights"

Small, two- or three-pound dumbbells are ideal, but that equipment is certainly not a requirement. You can choose virtually anything to add some weight to your routines, though you probably want to choose things you can easily hold in your hands, such as water bottles or food cans. Figure 20-1 shows these options.

REMEMBER

That's by no means an exhaustive list. As long as it's about two to three pounds, it fits in your hand, and you have at least two of it, any item will do.

Evaluating whether Yogic breathing with weights is right for you

Moving with your breath helps ensure you remain as relaxed as possible during your Yoga practice. As we explain in Chapter 3, the Yoga tradition most often says that you inhale (breathe in) when your body reaches or expands and you exhale (breathe out) when your body folds.

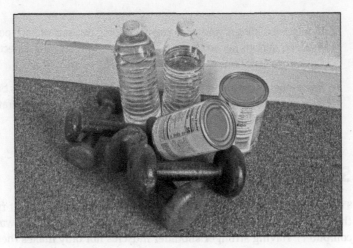

FIGURE 20-1:
Dumbbell
options.

The challenge when combining Yoga with weights, however, is that the best way to breathe may be different depending on whether you're also participating in another sport/working with a personal trainer.

TIP

Stay with what you know. If Yoga is your sole activity, stick with the Yoga-style breathing. If you're doing Yoga on top of another sport or activity that has you breathing another way, stick to that sport's method. The most important thing is just to keep breathing.

Using Weights in Chair Yoga

Sitting in a chair is a perfect place to grab some weights to add a little resistance work to your routine. The following sections provide a sampling of Chair Yoga poses that incorporate dumbbells.

REMEMBER

Keep in mind that the right amount of weight, as well as the number of repetitions in any routine, varies from person to person. Feel free to adjust anything in these exercises to better suit your particular body. And, as always, nothing you do should cause pain or discomfort beyond light muscle fatigue.

TIP

Here are a few suggestions to help you make the most of these poses:

>> If you don't think adding weight is appropriate for you, you can do these routines without weights (with empty hands). Though you may not get the added muscle-building benefits, the movements are still good for your joints and overall flexibility.

>> If muscle-building *is* your goal, consider doing two sets of each pose, and/or more repetitions per set, to enhance the strength-building aspects of this Chair Yoga variation.

>> Remember that other movements we describe throughout this book may also allow you to add weights. The following examples are just inspirations, not a complete list of every pose you can do with weights.

Shoulder shrugs with weights

This routine targets your shoulder muscles, which can get tight from so much of the routine movement you do (whether it's driving on the freeway or sitting at a computer). Having stronger shoulder muscles not only makes these routine tasks easier but also helps your overall posture. You can read more about Chair Yoga for your shoulders in Chapter 6.

1. **Sitting tall in your chair, grip your weights and let your arms hang straight down at your sides with your palms facing in (see Figure 20-2).**

2. **On an inhale, lift your shoulders up toward your ears, keeping your arms hanging (see Figure 20-3).**

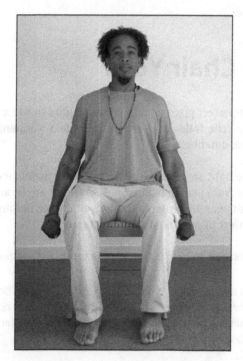

FIGURE 20-2: Starting position.

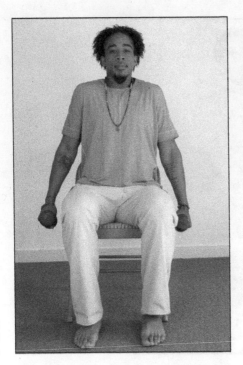

FIGURE 20-3:
Shrugging with
weights.

3. As you exhale, lower your shoulders back to your starting position.

4. Repeat Steps 1 through 3 for a total of 10 to 15 reps.

Bicep curls

Aside from looking good in a sleeveless shirt, strong biceps provide general support for your shoulders and the rest of your upper body.

1. Sitting tall in your chair, with both feet on the ground (or a prop), grip your weights comfortably on your thighs with your palms facing up (see Figure 20-4).

2. On an exhale, bend your arms as you bring the weights up toward you (see Figure 20-5).

3. As you inhale, lower your hands back down to your starting position.

4. Repeat Steps 1 through 3 for a total of 10 to 15 reps.

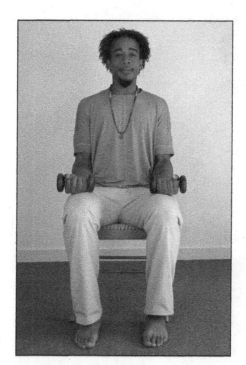

FIGURE 20-4:
Starting position.

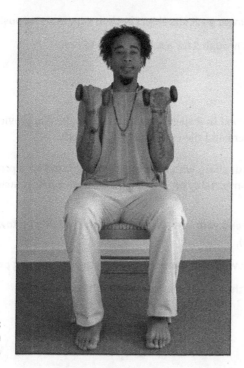

FIGURE 20-5:
Bicep curls with
weights.

Triceps pulses

Strong *triceps* (the backs of your upper arms) not only enhance the overall fitness of your upper body but also make routine lifting tasks easier.

1. **Sit tall in your chair with your arms hanging straight down, gripping your weights with your palms facing inward (see Figure 20-6).**

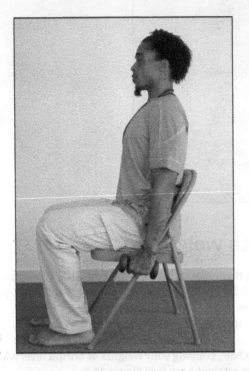

FIGURE 20-6:
Starting position.

2. **Lean forward (hinging from the hips) and raise your straight arms behind you until you feel some natural resistance.**

3. **Without holding your breath, pulse your arms upward, feeling the tension in the back of your upper arms (see Figure 20-7).**

4. **Continue to pulse, breathing normally, for about five breaths.**

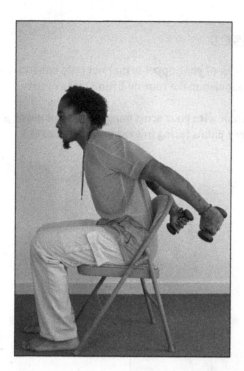

FIGURE 20-7:
Triceps pulses
with weights.

Rowing with weights

Generally speaking, rowing exercises are good all-around routines that target the whole body. From your chair, you're particularly focusing on your back (upper back and the muscles between your shoulder blades). Of course, imagining you're in a rowboat on a quiet lake may make this routine even easier.

1. Sit tall in your chair, gripping your weights at armpit level with, with your elbows pointing straight back (see Figure 20-8).

2. On an inhale, extend your arms straight out in front of you (see Figure 20-9).

3. As you exhale, bend your elbows and come back to the starting position.

4. Repeat Steps 1 through 3 for a total of eight to ten reps.

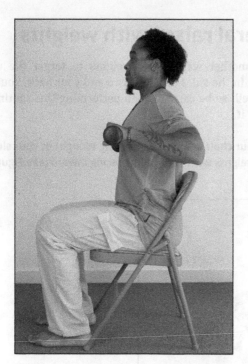

FIGURE 20-8:
Starting position.

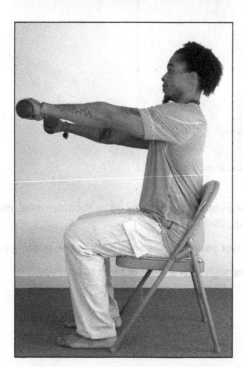

FIGURE 20-9:
Rowing with weights.

Seated lateral raises with weights

Lateral raises are another way to use weights to target the upper body — particularly muscles in the sides of your torso and your back. Your shoulders are going to feel it as well, so be careful when performing this routine. If it bothers your shoulders, skip it.

1. Sitting tall in your chair, let your arms hang straight at your sides, gripping your weights with your palms facing inward (see Figure 20-10).

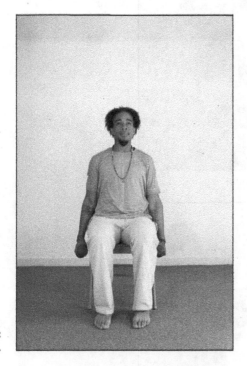

FIGURE 20-10:
Starting position.

2. On an inhale, bring your straight arms up to shoulder level, making a T-shape (see Figure 20-11).

3. As you exhale, lower your straight arms back to the starting position.

4. Repeat Steps 1 through 3 for a total of eight to ten reps.

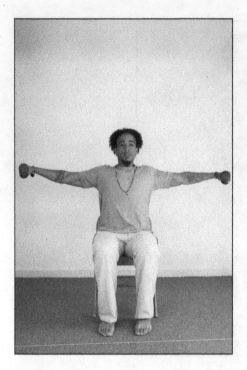

FIGURE 20-11:
Arms in a
T-shape.

Seated twists with weights

With or without weights, Yoga traditionally sees twists as being very detoxifying. Stretching the muscles around the waist and back may be the biggest modern-day benefit. You want to have that range of motion when you suddenly turn around from behind the wheel of a car to reach something in the back seat. A flexible waist and back help prevent an injury or tweak.

1. Sit tall in your chair, gripping the weights so that they're resting just above your shoulders (see Figure 20-12).

2. Inhale; on your exhale, rotate your torso all the way to the left.

3. On your inhale, rotate back to the center.

4. On your exhale, rotate your torso all the way to the right (see Figure 20-13).

5. Repeat Steps 2 through 4, following your breath, for a total of eight to ten reps.

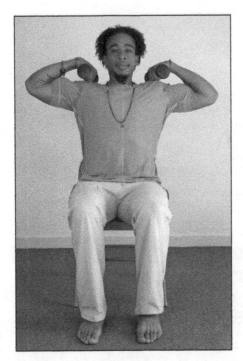

FIGURE 20-12:
Starting position.

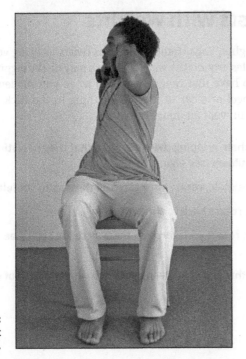

FIGURE 20-13:
Seated twist
with weights.

Heel lifts with weights

For this routine, the target is your legs — with particular focus on the calves. Do one leg at a time so that you can add more weight resistance.

1. **Sit tall in your chair; gripping a weight in each hand, place both weights on your right thigh with your palms facing down (see Figure 20-14).**

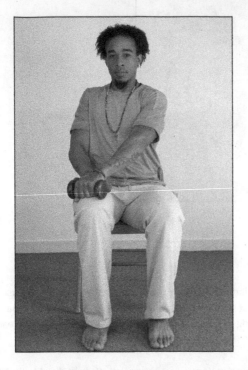

FIGURE 20-14:
Starting position.

2. **On an inhale, lift your right heel as high as you can without lifting your right toes (see Figure 20-15).**

3. **As you exhale, lower your heel back to the starting position.**

4. **Repeat Steps 1 through 3 for one to two minutes.**

   You can keep going for longer, if needed; just stop before your calf starts to cramp.

5. **Repeat Steps 1 through 4 on the other side.**

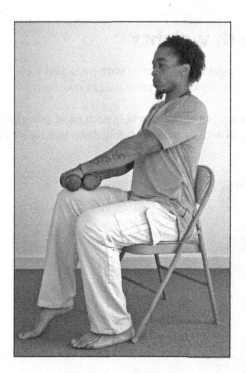

FIGURE 20-15:
Heel lifts.

BULK TALK

Back in the 1950s, the famous body builder, Charles Atlas, flexed his muscles in the pages of America's most popular newspapers and magazines. And probably since then, people have been asking if using weights — even in a Yoga class — will lead to an unwanted "bulking up." The answer is no.

Typically, the weights used in Yoga classes are relatively light dumbbells. This is certainly true with the Chair Yoga routines described in this chapter. The addition of weights into Chair Yoga may indeed demand more strength and endurance and ultimately yield even more fitness benefits. However, the chances that the added weight will be enough to actually build a significant amount of muscle mass is highly unlikely — especially if the dumbbells you choose are still light enough to ensure the integrity of your movements and the evenness of your breath.

So, rest assured that adding weights to some primary Yoga movements may ultimately lead to better muscle tone, improved cardiovascular health, or even higher bone density (depending on the expert you're consulting). What doesn't seem to be debatable is that Chair Yoga with manageable weights will not bulk you up — even if you want it to.

The Part of Tens

Chapter **21**

Ten Things to Remember about Chair Yoga

C hair Yoga should feel good; it should make you more energetic, stronger, and more flexible. It should improve your posture and maybe even the quality of your sleep.

If too much inactivity is one of today's biggest threats to health, Chair Yoga may be part of the remedy you need. So much depends on the choices you make as you embrace Chair Yoga, so please keep these ten points in mind.

It's Not That Easy

Sometimes people have a tendency to think of Chair Yoga as being some kind of "Yoga-lite" — a notion that couldn't be more untrue. Although Chair Yoga may accommodate certain practitioners' limitations, it still provides many of the benefits associated with Yoga.

In fact, using the chair as a prop may allow you to go even more deeply into a pose or find a new pose altogether. If you're knowledgeable about it, Chair Yoga can keep you practicing for a lifetime.

TIP

In some cases, working with a teacher who knows your personal limitations and can help adapt a practice just for you may be beneficial.

Simple Movement Is Powerful

As co-author Larry Payne always tells his students, "You don't have to do the hardest poses to get results." That's because even simple movements or basic poses offer great benefits. Some routines seem almost too rudimentary, but the simplest of movements actually help build muscles, increase elasticity, lubricate joints, and improve your mental outlook.

Don't Dangle

In Chair Yoga, you may find that your feet dangle instead of resting comfortably on the floor because the seat is just a bit too far off the ground. This posture is a problem for your spine and can even lead to back problems.

But rest easy; you don't have to search for a new chair. Instead, slide something underneath your feet to bring the floor up to you. A Yoga block or two work well, or you can use a stack of magazines, a box, or a pile of blankets. The goal is to allow your feet to sit securely on something, taking that dangling weight away.

Know When to Say When

An instinct common to most people says that if a little of something is good for your, a lot of that same thing must be even better. But it rarely is.

Even in Chair Yoga, a practice that by nature considers your limitations, proceeding with patience is important. Let your body get used to moving if that's not something you do regularly; let your mind grow accustomed to silence or stillness if that's unusual or atypical. And, most of all, stop if what you're doing hurts (as we discuss later in the chapter) or if some voice in the back of your head tells you, "Enough!" Stay healthy so you can practice again another day.

Comfort Is Always in Fashion

Like a warm blanket, a hot bath, or a long walk on a sunny day, a Chair Yoga session should be something that makes you feel good, or maybe just alive. If it becomes something to look forward to, you'll come back to it on a regular basis. And, as we point out throughout this book, consistency is the key to success.

You Don't Need a Lot of Space

Chair Yoga is inherently somewhat self-contained. You may be seated for an entire class.

TIP

You can do Chair Yoga in a very limited amount of space, including at your desk or from your seat in coach. Still, ideally you want to be sitting in a place that allows you to freely raise your arms (forward and sideways) or extend your legs outward.

Keep Breathing

One of your primary goals in Chair Yoga is to keep your breathing nice and easy. That's why you see so many breath cues.

Yoga sees a direct relationship between stress and the way you breathe. Rapid breathing or holding your breath sends a message to your nervous system that you need help. That assistance usually comes in the form of certain hormones, like adrenaline, that boost your metabolism (and your stress levels right along with it). The best way to prevent this spike is to keep breathing slowly, through only your nose if possible. You can read more about Yoga breathing in Chapter 3.

Make the Time

Like with most activities that offer potential health benefits, Chair Yoga is more effective when your routines are regular.

Practicing once will probably only make you a little sore. Practicing as part of a regimen allows both the physical and mental advantages to happen more quickly. Even if you already have a full schedule, see where you can incorporate Chair Yoga into your daily or weekly routine. Then stick to the plan.

Don't Let It Hurt

Chair Yoga may cause some soreness, but it shouldn't hurt. In Chair Yoga, pain signals are likely signs you're pushing too hard or going too deeply into a pose. (We talk more about the difference between soreness and pain in Chapter 15.)

REMEMBER

If you pay attention to pain signals and back off when necessary, you're protecting yourself against injury and demonstrating an ability to practice more advanced Yoga.

You Don't Have to Use the Chair Forever (But You Can)

Chair Yoga can serve two distinct roles in your life. If your limitations are temporary, practicing from a chair can be a great way to accommodate your injury or illness. At the appropriate time, you can then transition back to more traditional styles of Yoga.

If, however, you find that the permanent changes in your body require an equally permanent change in approach, Chair Yoga is something you can stick with on a regular basis. Whether your Chair Yoga practice is carved in stone or a stepping-stone, it can keep you moving and keep your breathing relaxed.

Chapter **22**

Ten Things to Do When Creating a Home Chair Yoga Practice

Reading about Chair Yoga is one thing. Incorporating it into your life is something else altogether.

Doing Chair Yoga at home is a challenge for any number of reasons, not the least of which is all the built-in distractions. Whether it's the telephone or TV, your pet or your family, you'll always have an unlimited number of commitments and chores to demand your attention and move Chair Yoga to the bottom of your to-do list.

REMEMBER

Part of you is always going to be looking for reasons not to practice. The health benefits of Chair Yoga are truly attainable when that practice is part of a regular routine.

If you've already convinced yourself that Chair Yoga would be a beneficial part of your life, the suggestions in this chapter may help you integrate that practice more easily.

Talk to Your Doctor

This may be standard advice before you start any type of fitness regime, but we want it to be more than a parenthetical warning here. Having a conversation with your doctor about your Chair Yoga plans lets you to better determine what your routine is going to look like. Your doctor may have some insights you don't have, so take the time to check in. For example, if your doctor says that your lower back problems stem from weak abdominal muscles, you may want to make sure your chair routine includes some strength work in that area.

WARNING

Your doctor can also highlight movements or postures, like forward bends or inversions, that you should definitely avoid because of preexisting conditions. For instance, twists can be dangerous if you've had certain joint replacements, and people who are pregnant or dealing with/at risk for osteoporosis should completely avoid certain poses.

Check Out Some Books and Videos

If you're practicing Chair Yoga at home and not getting in-person instruction, you're probably going to rely on books and/or videos. Both have their advantages and disadvantages:

>> **Books:** Books, especially hard-copy ones, typically require less technology. But you're limited to the photographs and text presented to give you direction.

>> **Videos:** Videos (DVDs or online clips) can show you an entire movement without needing a block of text to explain it. The downside is that where you practice is limited by factors like where your device can go and how reliable your Internet connection is.

Find the Right Expert

Because you have a plethora of Chair Yoga resources available to you, you have to be selective. One of the most important criteria for choosing a teacher is their level of knowledge. You want to find one who knows Chair Yoga and presents it in a way that is both accessible and safe. But don't discount the importance of finding a teacher who also resonates with you. Maybe you simply need to ask yourself whether you like the sound of their voice or the way they deliver instructions.

TIP

If you feel like you don't have the expertise to discern who is or isn't a good instructor, ask someone you trust for referrals the same way you would for a mechanic or a dentist.

Create a Dedicated Space

TIP

Find a place — a spot and a chair that you'll always use for your practice — ahead of time. You don't need a lot of space, and making this simple effort in advance can do a lot to keep your motivation intact.

As we discuss in the earlier "Check Out Some Books and Videos" section, technology constraints can limit your location choices. Scoping all that out ahead of time can help keep you from any surprises that spoil your enthusiasm.

Build Practice Time into Your Schedule

Chair Yoga fits perfectly into the extra time you have in your day, although most people don't have a lot of extra time. The key is to plan. Designating a certain hour of the day or maybe day of the week to devote to Chair Yoga allows you to integrate the practice more easily into your regular routine so it becomes automatic.

Set Expectations

Keep your expectations realistic, but feel free to adjust them along the way. Maybe initially, just scheduling your session and then doing it is your only goal. The consistency of your practice over time will allow you to consider more challenging goals like increasing flexibility and strength, reducing certain pain, or maybe even losing some weight.

REMEMBER

Whatever motivates you to begin a regular Chair Yoga regimen, don't let those motivations work against you. Give your practice time to yield results.

Invite a Friend

Practicing alone at home doesn't always have the social component you may find in a studio class, so you may want to consider inviting another person or people to join you. For some folks, the communal aspect of practicing with other people is another form of motivation — a shared experience that brings together like-minded people. Having other people involved can also be a way to hold you accountable and has its own health benefits.

Be Still and Breathe

Yoga has a concept of *constructive rest* that basically acknowledges the mental and physical benefits of simply doing nothing. In fact, most Yoga classes end with some variation of *savasana* (the Sanskrit name of a pose that translates to "corpse pose"). This resting pose gives the body a chance to rebuild and the mind a chance to relax.

In Chair Yoga, don't underestimate the value of taking a little time for breath work or meditation. Although at first you may feel like you're just sitting in your chair doing nothing, you're in fact repairing your body, reducing stress, and possibly fighting both mental and physical fatigue (if you're not getting the rest you need during sleep). Besides, it may be the most rest you get in the course of your day.

Meditate in Your Chair

Sitting in a chair is the perfect place to meditate, and you should consider it part of your Chair Yoga practice even if you choose to do it separately from the other chair routines. As we explain in Chapter 4, even practitioners at meditation centers sometimes opt for a chair.

REMEMBER

Meditation shouldn't be painful. You shouldn't be distracted by the discomfort of sitting on the floor or the prospect of getting down and then back up. If sitting in your chair allows you to focus more on what's happening internally rather than the external pain or discomfort, you're truly ahead of the game.

Keep It Fun

Chair Yoga needs to be something you do on a regular basis, and you'll have better luck making it part of your routine if you keep it fun. Maybe that means including music as part of your session, or perhaps other people. (Head to the earlier section "Invite a Friend" for more on that.) Ultimately, it's up to you. It won't be an enjoyable experience if you encounter pain, so don't do anything so long that it hurts.

Index

barefoot, 131–132

"bat wings," 121

Beginner routines, 168–171, 176–184

Belly Breathing exercise, 36–37, 184

Bent Knee Lifts exercise, 89–90

Bent Leg Arm Raise exercise, 168

Bicep Curls exercise, 219–220

biceps, 112

body parts, used in breathing, 32–33

bone density
  as a benefit of Yoga, 12
  increasing with weighted Chair Yoga, 216

bones, in ankles and feet, 124–125

books
  reading, 20–21
  as resources, 236

Breath Awareness meditation, 47

Breath-Focused meditation, 42

breathing
  about, 29–30
  alternate nostril, 37–40
  belly, 36–37
  benefits of, 29
  body parts used in, 32–33
  Chair Yoga and, 233, 238
  focus, 35–36
  importance of, 30–32
  managing stress and pain with, 34–40
  as a principle of practice, 162
  problems with, 34
  relationship with posture, 30, 32

sleep and, 31

weighted Chair Yoga and, 216–217

bursitis, elbows and, 113

C

calf muscles, 104

carpal tunnel syndrome, 134, 135

Chair Thunderbolt Variation exercise, 201–203

Chair Yoga
  for abdominals, 88–94
  about, 7–8, 145, 161
  adding meditation to, 41–49
  adding weights to, 215–228
  for ankles, 125–131
  for the back, 77–83
  benefits of, 7
  breathing and, 233, 238
  clothing for, 22
  creating a practice, 235–239
  at a desk, 193–205
  difficulty level for, 231–232
  dynamic/static approach, 163
  for feet, 125–131
  for fingers, 135–144
  forgiving limbs, 163–164
  for hands, 135–144
  for hips, 98–102
  inversion poses and, 147–158
  for legs, 106–110
  location for, 21–22, 233, 237
  meditation and, 238
  mindset for, 164

H

Half Forward Fold with a Chair
    exercise, 148
hamstrings, 104
hands
  about, 133
  arthritis and, 134
  Chair Yoga for, 135–144
  median nerve, 135
  mudras, 144
  preventing pain and stiffness in, 133–135
head rolls, 56
heart, inversion poses and, 147
heart chakra (anahata), 44
Heel Lifts with Weights exercise, 227–228
height, of chairs, 23–24, 232
Hip Circles exercise, 98–99, 170, 179
hip flexors, 95
hips
  about, 95
  caring for, 95–98
  Chair Yoga for, 98–102
  emotions and, 98
  opening your, 96
  preventing injuries in, 96–97
Hirschi, Gertrude
  Mudras: Yoga in Your Hands, 144
hot spots, 194–195

I

icons, explained, 3
injuries
  elbows and, 113
  preventing in hips, 96–97

I

Instinctive Meditation (IM), 42
intercostal muscles, 30
Inversion: Legs on a Chair exercise,
    157–158
inversion poses
  about, 146–148
  adding chairs to, 145–158
  Chair Yoga and, 147–158
Iyengar, B.K.S. (Yoga master), 1, 9, 18,
    145, 165

J

joint lubrication
  as a benefit of Yoga, 11
  Chair Yoga for, 134
Jois, K. Pattabi, 165

K

kinetic chain, 124
Knee Circles exercise, 169
Knee to Elbow exercise, 211–212
knees, 104–105
Krishnamacharya, Tirumalai, 40, 165

L

legs
  about, 103–104
  Chair Yoga for, 106–110
  cramps, 106
  knees, 104–105
limited mobility, Chair Yoga for people
    with, 10
location, for Chair Yoga, 21–22, 233, 237
Loving/Kindness meditation, 42–43

O

One Leg Forward Bend exercise, 173
One Leg Hamstring stretch, 181
opening your hips, 96
osteoporosis, 124

P

pain
  about, 164
  Chair Yoga and, 232, 234
  in hands, fingers, and wrists, 133–135
parasympathetic nervous system, 31
Patanjali
  Yoga Sutras, 31–32
Payne, Larry (author), 15, 18, 40, 165,
    213, 232
  Yoga For Dummies, 1
physical breaks, Chair Yoga at desks for,
    193–194
poses
  Chair Yoga Boat pose, 190
  Chair Yoga Tree pose (standing), 191
  inversion poses, 145–158
  Seated Warrior One pose, 106–108
  Seated Warrior Two pose, 108, 109
posture
  abdominal work and, 86–87
  relationship with breathing, 30, 32
  sitting up straight, 67
  sitting with good, 88–89
practice, principles of, 161–164
pranayama, 42
prayer meditation, 43

Prime of Life Yoga (POLY), 15, 62–64, 165
principles of practice, 161–164

Q

quadricep, 104

R

Ramaswami, Srivatsa, 165
real-time classes, 20
Rejuvenation Sequence, 15
relaxation, inversion poses and, 147
Remember icon, 3
repetitive stress injuries, 134
rest, in Beginner routine, 171
Roche, Lorin, 42
root chakra (muladhara), 44
Rounding Shoulders exercise, 66–67
routines
  Advanced, 171–174, 184–192
  Beginner, 168–171, 176–184
  fifteen-minute, 167–174
  thirty-minute, 175–192
Rowing with Weights exercise, 222–223

S

sacral chakra (svadhisthana), 44
Seated Bicep Curls with Weights
    exercise, 188
Seated Boat Pose exercise, 90–91
Seated Camel exercise, 83, 179
Seated Cat/Cow exercise, 79–81,
    176–177
Seated Flies exercise, 189

Larry Payne, PhD, C-IAYT, E-RYT500, is an internationally respected Yoga teacher, author, and a founding father of Yoga therapy in America. Dr. Payne cofounded the International Association of Yoga Therapists, now in 50 countries, and the Yoga curriculum at the UCLA School of Medicine. He is also the founder of the Yoga Therapy Rx and Prime of Life Yoga programs at Loyola Marymount University (LMU), the corporate Yoga program at the J. Paul Getty Museum, and the original "Back Program" at the world-famous Rancho La Puerta Fitness Spa.

In 2000, he was the first Yoga teacher to be invited to the World Economic Forum in Davos, Switzerland, and in 1996, he performed the first documented headstand at the North Pole with the World Presidents' Organization (WPO). He founded Samata International Yoga and Health Center in Los Angeles in 1980, where he continues to teach groups and individuals.

Dr. Payne is coauthor of the international bestseller *Yoga For Dummies* and *Yoga Basics* (both published by Wiley), *Yoga Rx* (Broadway Books), *The Business of Teaching Yoga* (Samata International), and *Yoga Therapy and Integrative Medicine* (Basic Health Publications, Inc). He is featured in the *Prime of Life Yoga* and *Yoga Therapy Rx* DVD series (available at Samata.com) and is featured globally online at Yoga International, Glo, and Yoga Download. Most recently, he authored AARP's *Yoga After 50 For Dummies* (Wiley). His website is Samata.com.

Don Henry, MA, C-IAYT, E-RYT500, is a long-time student of Larry's, a graduate of LMU's Yoga therapy program (Levels I–IV), and a certified Yoga therapist (featured in *HuffPost*). Additionally, Don studied one-on-one with American Chair Yoga pioneer Lakshmi Voelker and is a certified LVCY Chair Yoga teacher. Don also completed three levels of Larry's Prime of Life Yoga (POLY) training and is a POLY-certified teacher. Most recently, he went through a 200-hour program in meditation taught by Lorin Roche and Camille Maurine and is now certified to teach Instinctive Meditation.

Continuing to work with Larry on a number of ongoing projects, Don also lectures and mentors in LMU's Yoga therapy program, teaches three public classes a week, and sees patients privately. His website is ageofyoga.com.

Dedication

Larry wants to dedicate this book to his lifelong friend, Merry Aronson.

Don dedicates this book to Lisa, his wife, who is now and has always been his biggest fan and most ardent supporter. He gives special thanks to Shanna Hughes who introduced him to Chair Yoga. He also wants to give his deepest appreciation to both Larry Payne, his dear friend and mentor, and also to his first Yoga teacher, Nicole Sciacca, for kindling his Yoga passion.

Authors' Acknowledgments

First, we want to thank Dr. Matthew Taylor for his technical review of this work. Our book has definitely benefited from his knowledge and insight.

We also want to thank Tracy Boggier at Wiley for initially supporting this project, and then Kelsey Baird, Chrissy Guthrie, Kristie Pyles, and Megan Knoll. They each helped to make the book development process a pleasure.

Of course, we are extremely grateful to Dr. Loren Fishman for writing the Foreword to this book. His encouragement and support have truly been inspirational.

Also, a great deal of appreciation goes to our Chair Yoga models: Alexis Estwick, Charles Fantroy, Traci Fantroy, Jerry Gil, Laura Liu, Chris Payne, Karen Perez, Candice Rosales, Teri Roseman, Ashley Smaldino, Melvin Stakely, Mandvi Tandon, Paula Tapia, and Sasi Velupillai. Many thanks to our talented hair and makeup artist, Mana Afshar.

Publisher's Acknowledgments

Associate Editor: Kelsey Baird

Project Manager and Development Editor: Christina N. Guthrie

Managing Editor: Kristie Pyles

Copy Editor: Megan Knoll

Technical Editor: Matthew J. Taylor, PhD

Production Editor: Saikarthick Kumarasamy

Cover Photos: Courtesy of Don Henry and Gavin DiPaola

Take dummies with you everywhere you go!

Whether you are excited about e-books, want more from the web, must have your mobile apps, or are swept up in social media, dummies makes everything easier.

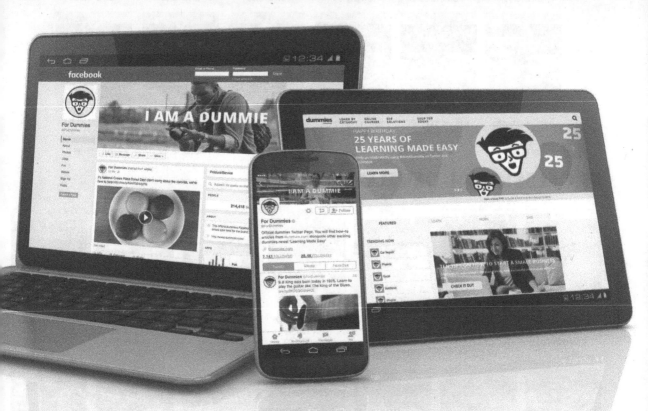

Find us online!

dummies.com

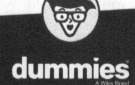

PERSONAL ENRICHMENT

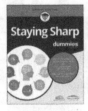
Staying Sharp
9781119187790
USA $26.00
CAN $31.99
UK £19.99

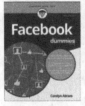
Facebook
9781119179030
USA $21.99
CAN $25.99
UK £16.99

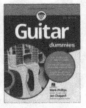
Guitar
9781119293354
USA $24.99
CAN $29.99
UK £17.99

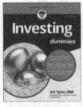
Investing
9781119293347
USA $22.99
CAN $27.99
UK £16.99

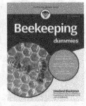
Beekeeping
9781119310068
USA $22.99
CAN $27.99
UK £16.99

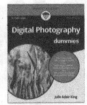
Digital Photography
9781119235606
USA $24.99
CAN $29.99
UK £17.99

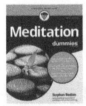
Meditation
9781119251163
USA $24.99
CAN $29.99
UK £17.99

Pregnancy
9781119235491
USA $26.99
CAN $31.99
UK £19.99

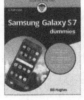
Samsung Galaxy S7
9781119279952
USA $24.99
CAN $29.99
UK £17.99

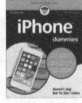
iPhone
9781119283133
USA $24.99
CAN $29.99
UK £17.99

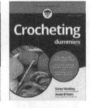
Crocheting
9781119287117
USA $24.99
CAN $29.99
UK £16.99

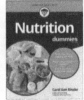
Nutrition
9781119130246
USA $22.99
CAN $27.99
UK £16.99

PROFESSIONAL DEVELOPMENT

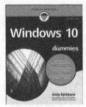
Windows 10
9781119311041
USA $24.99
CAN $29.99
UK £17.99

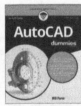
AutoCAD
9781119255796
USA $39.99
CAN $47.99
UK £27.99

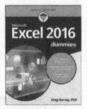
Excel 2016
9781119293439
USA $26.99
CAN $31.99
UK £19.99

QuickBooks 2017
9781119281467
USA $26.99
CAN $31.99
UK £19.99

macOS Sierra
9781119280651
USA $29.99
CAN $35.99
UK £21.99

LinkedIn
9781119251132
USA $24.99
CAN $29.99
UK £17.99

Windows 10 All-in-One
9781119310563
USA $34.00
CAN $41.99
UK £24.99

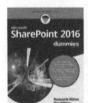
SharePoint 2016
9781119181705
USA $29.99
CAN $35.99
UK £21.99

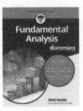
Fundamental Analysis
9781119263593
USA $26.99
CAN $31.99
UK £19.99

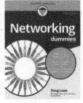
Networking
9781119257769
USA $29.99
CAN $35.99
UK £21.99

Office 2016
9781119293477
USA $26.99
CAN $31.99
UK £19.99

Office 365
9781119265313
USA $24.99
CAN $29.99
UK £17.99

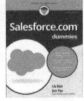
Salesforce.com
9781119239314
USA $29.99
CAN $35.99
UK £21.99

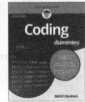
Coding
9781119293323
USA $29.99
CAN $35.99
UK £21.99